Triage, Trauma, and Drama

Copyright © 2023 by Matthew Burkey-Gilchrist

All rights reserved.

No portion of this book may be reproduced in any form without written permission from the publisher or author, except as permitted by U.S. copyright law.

Contents

1. Triage, Trauma, And Drama — 1
2. Rules of EMS — 4
3. It's Just Richard — 7
4. Dangerous Words — 13
5. My P**** — 20
6. Crash — 26
7. Burn — 32
8. Clear! — 39
9. Judge and Jury — 45
10. Say What — 51
11. I Know — 57
12. Why To Hide Your Lube — 61
13. Implied Consent — 66
14. One With The Force — 74
15. Stories From Triage — 79
16. Squirrel In The Box — 89

17. Shit Magnets   95

18. Nope, Still Dead   104

Chapter One

Triage, Trauma, And Drama

Dedicated to my Uncle David

Honestly, I never really thought that this book would get written. For years, everyone has been telling me I really need to write this stuff down, just in case I someday forgot it. I'm not sure if it's a blessing or a curse, but I remember most of these stories in this book in very vivid detail. I can still recall all their faces and all their names. So, forgetting is not something that I'm likely to do.

Why I'm writing it now, I guess I finally feel like some of these stories are old enough to be told. And recent familial events have given me a stark reminder that we may have as long on this earth as we thought we did. I've altered names, places, and some details just to make them generic enough that anyone could come across them in the field or the hospital. There are no real names used, aside from my own.

I have been an EMS professional for 21 years now. When I started off in this career field, I had never imagined that it would take me to some places it has. If you had told twenty-one-year-old me I would someday end up in a helicopter, then I probably would have laughed in your face. I also would have pointed out how terrified I was of being in a helicopter. To this day, I'm still surprised they got me up in one.

This profession has been one of highs and lows for me. I love what I do, but to say that it has always been smooth sailing would be a flat-out lie. Although rewarding, this career has left its scars on me. It has cost me relationships and time spent with loved ones. I've seen the best and worst that humanity can do to each other in a few hours. I've seen the beauty of new life and the peace of death. There were days I got home from work and just cried. There were a few days when I even considered never going back again.

And just when I feel like I'm tapped out, I somehow come back for more. Maybe we're all just gluttons for punishment. I'd like to think it's more than that, though, that we have this innate instinct to help our fellow man. We may not always do it with a smile, but we always put our patients before ourselves. It takes a certain breed to work in this profession. Sometimes those that feel the most broken are the best at healing others, born out of a lifetime of experiencing some kind of pain.

The pandemic has revealed the extraordinary character of healthcare workers, and their vulnerability to burnout, fatigue, and mental health issues. I'm not immune to those factors. I'm still dealing with twenty years of repressed trauma and seeing things that I have never really processed. Know that you aren't alone in that battle, trust me. We've all faced that struggle, even if we don't want to admit it.

I have done 911, Critical Care Transport, Not So Critical Transport, and Flight Medicine. I have had the distinct pleasure of serving with some of the best EMTs, nurses, and medics in the field. We're an odd fraternity of trauma junkies that operate on tiny amounts of sleep and high amounts of caffeine. This isn't just a job for most of us. It's a calling and a way to serve our fellow man. Lord knows we don't do it for the pay.

The stories inside are humorous, tragic, and sometimes downright depressing. Because that's what medicine is. We don't have all the answers. We don't save everyone and people will stay die despite all our efforts and technology. Sometimes we feel ashamed that we couldn't save the person or maybe guilty that our training didn't provide us with the knowledge to combat death.

And that's okay, just so long as you know that no matter what you do, people will still die. It's not a prospect that I liked to think about when I was first starting off in this career, but now, at twenty years in, one that often crosses my mind. Especially in the wee hours of the morning as I am pushing on a person's chest.

I hate the saying 'doing battle with the grim reaper'. I know that when I was a young, dumb paramedic, I wore shirts that said that. Hell, I probably even said it on more than one occasion. What we do every day is to heal, to serve life, to preserve it. Believe me, if whatever deity you believe in exists and they are our calling that soul home, there isn't a damn thing that we mortals are going to do about it. So, cut yourself some slack.

I hope that what you are about to read makes you laugh, smile, and maybe even reflect a little. So, sit back and enjoy Triage, Trauma, and Drama.

Chapter Two

Rules of EMS

EMS professionals and ER staff are a superstitious lot. There are certain words that you should never utter in our presence, lest you anger the gods and bring down wrath upon us all. If you think that I'm kidding, walk into an ER sometime and say 'Gee, it's quiet in here.' Go ahead, I dare you. You'll be lucky to make it out of there alive. EMS has an entirely unique set of rules and breaking any of these cardinal rules is an invitation for the Gods of Motorola to rain down their wrath on the unsuspecting squads.

#1. Sick people don't bitch. When people are truly hurting, they aren't complaining about how cold the ambulance is, what the radio station is on, or how bored they are during the ride. Sick people just want to lie there and do nothing.

#2. Air goes in and out, blood goes round and round. Any variation on this is a bad thing. Blood covering the floor of your ambulance or ER bay is bad. Air coming out of anywhere but your nose or mouth, is also bad.

#3. When dealing with patients, supervisors, or citizens, if it felt good saying it, it was the wrong thing to say. We've all been guilty of breaking this rule at least once in our careers. At least, I have. I've uttered such things as 'shark attack' (at a person's home, in a landlocked state) or 'his flux capacitor broke' to citizens that kept asking what was going on during scene calls.

#4. All bleeding stops... eventually.

#5. It is bad to use the words "holy shit" regarding the patient's condition. I'm sure, as you'll soon find out, I have violated this rule on multiple occasions. I try not to make it obvious, but sometimes you just have to say it. There are certain situations that warrant such a response, despite what management says.

#6. When responding to a call, always remember that the lowest bidder built your ambulance.

#7. Uttering the Q word (quiet) while in the presence of emergency personnel will cause an immediate and swift beating. Well, probably not really, but you will make emergency personnel incredibly upset. You may also cause the ER and or your service area of your ambulance to suddenly encounter the most fucked up shit that you have ever seen. And great numbers of fucked up shit.

#8. People don't call an ambulance or to the ER because they did something right. If you're new to EMS or working in an emergency room, this is often one of the hardest things to remember. No one is calling the ambulance or coming to the ER after doing something intelligent. Most ER trips or calls to emergency services start off with that little-known phrase "Here, hold my beer."

#9. There will be no dying or multiplying in the back of my unit. Birthing does not happen in the back of my ambulance. Dying does not happen in the back of my ambulance. You will end the call with the EXACT number of patients that you started the call with. We don't add patients or subtract them. And no one dies in the back of the ambulance either, you do that shit at the hospital.

#10. It's the patient's emergency, not yours. You've been trained for this, and even if you haven't, you better damn well make sure it looks like you have. Keep calm, take a deep breath, and use your head. Losing your cool will not make the situation any better.

#11. Asystole is a stable rhythm. No, you didn't read that wrong. You can't get more dead than dead. In fact, your condition can only improve, not get any worse.

#12. Everyone was new at this once…despite what they say. No one was born holding trauma sheers and with the ability to hit every vein, every time, no matter what they say. We all had to start somewhere. You're going to make mistakes and that's okay. It's called learning, it's what adults do. And sometimes you're going to have to learn things the hard way. That's okay too.

Chapter Three

It's Just Richard

One thing that I really enjoyed about working in EMS is the chance to build relationships with the community that you serve. Working in the field is a great way to expose yourself to new viewpoints and cultures. I learned a lot from working with people of various races, religions, and minorities.

One downside about working in the field is that you meet lots of what we call frequent flyers. These are the people that call EMS or that show up at the ER so much that they know the staff by name. I encountered one such frequent flyer by the name of Richard (not his real name). The first time that I met Richard, he was throwing himself off the roof of his one-story garage onto his grass. The fall was approximately eight feet and Richard was about six two.

Now, to be fair, the first three times that we had been called for this, we treated it like it was a genuine cry for help. At least until we got to the hospital. Where he would tear his c-collar off, stand up, and declare himself healed by the aura of the hospital. He would rip off the collar, get out of the cot, and usually run off into the night.

Since then, every single time that we were called to his address, we'd find the same thing. Richard, half-naked, running across the roof of his garage and then falling off the edge onto the grass. He would then pop back to his feet, climb up a ladder and then do the whole thing all over again. Usually, it took us a few times to convince him he needed to go to the hospital or at least get in the ambulance.

On this fall afternoon, we had a student with us. I remember the terror that went along with being a student. When they were assigned to me, I tried not to be as big an asshole as some of my preceptors had been to me. So, when the call came out to 43 Birch Street, I had to repress the grin on my face. Mostly because this student was wound so tight that if you stuck a piece of coal up his ass, he'd be able to produce a diamond in mere minutes.

We pulled up to the curb just as Richard was falling off the roof. He hit the ground, lay there for a minute, and then popped back up and ran back around toward the ladder that was propped up against the side of the garage.

The student was running around the back of the ambulance to grab the backboard and trauma bag, while I and my partner slowly walked toward Richard. We were halfway there when he fell off the roof again. Once again, he lay there for a few seconds before popping back up and scrambling around to the ladder again.

"Do you want to stop him this time?" I asked.

My partner shrugged. By the time he got to the roof again, the students arrived with both the backboard and trauma bag. He gave a startled yelp when Richard fell off the roof again, landing just a few feet from us. I looked at my partner and then we both looked back down at Richard as he opened his eyes again. He glanced up at us, while the medic student just kind of stood there in shock.

"Am I dead?"

"No."

"So, I'm not in heaven?"

"Wait, you aren't going to do anything?" the student asked.

My partner held up his hand. "In a minute."

"No Richard, you aren't in heaven."

"Are you sure?"

I exhaled loudly. "Yes, Richard I'm sure."

"Okay."

"Did you take your meds today?" my partner asked.

"No."

"Did you take your meds at all this week?" I asked.

Richard thought about it for a second before shaking his head. "No, I don't think I have."

"Do you still have your meds?"

"Um, maybe? Should I try one more time before we go to the hospital?"

"I don't think so. You're making our paramedic student very nervous right now."

"Oh, okay."

The student who had dropped the backboard looked back and forth between us and Richard.

"Um, what should I do?" he asked.

"You should probably put the c-collar on me," Richard said. "And then you need to get me on the backboard."

The medic student looked at us and then back down at Richard.

"Well?" I asked. "What are you waiting for?"

Five minutes later, we had him loaded up and in the back of the ambulance.

"Shouldn't we start an IV?" the student asked.

I shrugged. "I dunno, Richard. Do you need an IV?"

"No, I'll be okay."

"Aren't they going to get mad if we bring in a trauma without at least one IV?" the student asked.

"Just tell them I wasn't cooperating," Richard said.

"Um, I don't think that I can do that," the student said.

"Sure you can," Richard said. He then motioned to me. "He does it all the time."

"That's not true."

"It is too."

"You put an IV in and he's just going to rip it out once we get there," my partner yelled from upfront.

The medic student took one look at me back down to Richard and then back at me again. He kind of looked like a deer caught in the headlights, not really sure what to do.

I just shrugged my shoulders. "He's your patient. Do what you feel is right."

"I really preferred if you did not start an IV," Richard said. "Like he said, I'm just going to rip it out when I get to the hospital."

I could practically see the smoke coming out of the medic students' ears. We're always taught that trauma patients get two large boar IVs. To show up at the hospital with none of that was blasphemy. It was the breaking of the Almighty trauma protocol. When I was a student, I lived and died by these rules.

I knew Richard wouldn't mind either way, but I was trying to get the student to focus on the overall picture, not just what he had seen. But, since he was a student, he still hadn't developed all his critical thinking skills yet. So he got out the IV bag and put two large bore IVs into Richard's arms.

I just shook my head and when I glanced up front, I could see my partner doing the same thing. We both knew exactly what was going to happen when we arrived at the hospital. I let the medic student give a report over the radio. I knew that everyone at the ER would know exactly who we were bringing in just by the report. That and they listen in to all the radio traffic between EMS and dispatch. Once we arrived at the hospital, my partner backed us smoothly into a parking place. Richard was relatively silent until we got out of the ambulance and started bringing him into the building.

As soon as we were inside the building, he sat up, ripped the c-collar off his neck, pulled out his IVs, and then jumped off the cot. And then Richard was off, screaming at the top of his lungs that we saved him, and then disappeared into the night. The medic student looked at me and then back at the fleeing shape of Richard.

"How are you guys okay with this?" he asked.

"It's sort of just what he does."

The student shook his head again. "I knew I would see some crazy things in EMS, but I guess I kind of thought some of those stories were wildly exaggerated."

I nodded. "I'm sure some of them are. However, with Richard, it's an actual thing."

"Isn't the hospital going to get mad?" he asked.

"Nah, after the report you gave, I'm pretty sure they knew exactly who it was already."

"Really?" he asked.

"Really, we'll go in and tell them what happened. Nothing will surprise them, trust me. Especially if it's Richard. We'll finish our report and go back into service."

"There are a lot of Richards in the world," my partner said. "You just need to learn to deal with them."

"I guess that's true," he said. "My classmates will never believe this."

I winked at him. "Do me a favor and don't tell anyone about it. Sometimes I'd like for them to have the same surprise that you did."

12

He laughed and nodded. "Sounds like a plan."

Chapter Four

Dangerous Words

WARNING: This chapter contains discussions of suicide.

I've been on my fair share of mental health calls in EMS. I've also taken care of plenty of patients in the ER that have mental health issues. They've run the gambit from depression and anxiety to full-blown schizophrenia. Dealing with patients that are suffering from a mental health crisis is never easy and can often make us feel uncomfortable as healthcare providers. The bottom line is that patients that are in the midst of a mental healthcare crisis still deserve the same amount of treatment as someone suffering from a heart attack.

My own personal experiences with suicide and depression certainly gave me more insight than some of my colleagues. I could understand what these people were going through. I had been there at one point in my own life, so I could understand the feelings of despair, hopelessness, and sadness that often took hold in those situations.

Don't get me wrong, we all know there are patients that exhibit attention-seeking behavior, but the vast majority of people seeking treatment for mental healthcare issues, are in genuine need. This story takes me back to one of the most intense attempts that I had seen.

your time in medicine, you develop a gut instinct. I always joke that I can feel a disturbance in the force. Although, that might be because I am just one huge Star Wars nerd. On this cloudy day (because it seems like this shit always happens on cloudy days), I woke up with an odd sense of dread. That happened occasionally, as someone that suffers from anxiety, I tried not to give it a second thought.

Usually, I could shake this kind of thing off. It would dissipate during my morning routine and eventually be gone by the time I arrived at the station. But it was still there when I got to work. Again, I thought after I got my rig checked, it would disappear. No such luck. It was even there after lunchtime, which is when I became convinced that something horrible was about to happen.

"You're doing that thing," my partner said.

"What thing?"

"That thing where you sense a disturbance in the force, don't you?"

I just shrugged and he rolled his eyes and let the matter drop. The call came in about a half hour later. A seventeen-year-old male was in his bathroom and not answering the door. His parents got concerned when he wouldn't answer the door or his friend's phone calls. The minute that we started rolling, I knew this was going to be a shit call. I could feel it in my gut.

We arrived at the same time as the fire and police departments. His mother was crying hysterically while his father just kept pounding on the door, yelling his name repeatedly. One policeman was in the middle of trying to talk to Mom when the FD made entry and then promptly yelled at us to get in there. We wasted no time in muscling our way around the officers and parents.

I stepped into the bathroom just as they were pulling a very pale and soaked body from the tub. The water in the bathtub was red, and it was then that I noticed two massive lacerations on the kid's forearms. These were not hesitant, shallow, horizontal cuts. These were deep vertical lacerations in arm, each a few inches long. As a pair of firefighters hauled him out of the bathtub, I heard his mom scream. The sound of a mother screaming always cuts me to the core. It's a kind of scream that sounds like nothing else.

What made the situation even worse was the fact that I couldn't even see any more blood coming from the wounds. How long had the poor kid been in there? Why the fuck didn't his parents call sooner? This was a serious attempt, a far cry from the kids that threatened to hurt themselves when they got grounded.

"He still has a pulse, but it's pretty weak and slow," one firefighter said.

They went to work cutting off his shirt and pants so that we could look for other wounds.

"Get us some towels," my partner snapped.

"What's his name?" I asked.

"Kevin," one policeman said.

"Kevin, can you hear me? I need you to open your eyes for me. Can you do that?"

"Blood pressure is only sixty by palp, respirations at 12 and shallow, pulse ox is 88 percent, putting him on a non-rebreather mask."

"Get the BVM. I'm not giving him a lot of leeway."

All I got was a moan from him. I looked over at the monitor and saw that his heart rate was only fifty. It looked like a suicide attempt, so he could have ingested something as well. I pressed my knuckles into his chest and rubbed hard. Again, I barely got a response from him. The firefighters were bandaging the injuries to his arms, although neither laceration was still bleeding.

"Pulse ox is coming up," one firefighter said. "Ninety-two percent, still breathing pretty shallow."

"Are there any mediations in the house that he could have taken?" my partner asked. "Anything at all?"

"I had some pain pills from back surgery a few months ago," the dad said.

"Where are they?" my partner asked, as he placed an IV in the kid's left arm.

The dad disappeared down the hallway and came back a moment later with an empty bottle. The look on his face was one of abject horror. He went almost as pale as the teenager laying on the bathroom floor.

"This was almost full!"

"Told you to flush them!" the mother screamed.

My partner grabbed the bottle and looked at the label. "Hydrocodone."

"Fuck."

"Narcan?"

"Yeah," I said. "And let's start some fluid."

We injected a little of the reversal agent slowly and started running our normal saline in. He needed blood, but right now I just needed to get his BP up and see if I could get him to come around. My partner started a second line on his other arm, which at least caused him to flinch. That was better than the response we had been getting a few minutes ago.

"Let's get going."

When we secured him on the backboard, he moaned again, this time much louder, and kind of reached up toward the oxygen mask that was on his face. Not completely awake, but doing better than he was. At least we were making progress in the right direction. As soon as we were in the ambulance, we took off toward the nearest hospital, which was about five minutes away.

"What the hell would make a kid do this?" my partner asked.

"He told his dad that one of his friends was gay last week," a firefighter said. "Apparently, his dad said that if he found out any of his kids were gay, he'd kick them out of the house and never talk to him again. After that conversation, Kevin went upstairs and the next time they saw him was when we were pulling him out of the tub."

"What the fuck? Really?"

"Really," he said. "I mean, who the hell says that to their kid?"

I shook my head. I couldn't fathom hearing your own dad say something so homophobic. Kevin moaned again as we went over another bump and his eyes fluttered open for a moment.

I wished he was more coherent so that I could ask him if this attempt on his life was because he was gay. Did he say it was a friend that was coming out just to test the waters? Being a guy that was still firmly in the closet, I could understand why. I had sat in that dark place during more than one time in my life. I knew what it took to drag you down and how hard you had to get back out.

His eyes fluttered open again, cutting to each of us in the back of the ambulance. I could see the momentary burst of panic and put my hand on his shoulder. He relaxed back in the cot as soon as my hand made contact.

"Kevin, can you hear me?"

I got a weak nod in response. Good.

"Did you take all those pills? Did you take anything else?"

Kevin weakly shook his head and reached up to pull the mask off his face again. I gently pulled his hand back down. "We're going to leave that on there for a little while, okay?"

He seemed to understand and put his hands back down.

"Did you do this on purpose?" I asked. "Were you trying to hurt yourself?"

I hoped he might answer honestly, considering his parents weren't anywhere near us.

Slowly, he nodded. My gut twisted at that thought.

"And you're sure that you took nothing else? You won't get into trouble, but we need to know so that we can make sure we get you the right medications."

Again, he slowly shook his head.

"And did you take all those pills?" I asked.

"Most," he whispered. "Not all. Couldn't keep them down, I threw up some in the toilet."

"Was it a lot?"

"Kinda," Kevin said.

"Does anything hurt besides your arms?"

A shake of his head.

"Great, are you having trouble breathing? Any chest pain or dizziness."

"Dizzy," he croaked. "And my head hurts and I feel cold."

That wasn't surprising, considering what he went through. I looked over at the monitor. His pulse ox was up to 97% and his heart rate had come up to the mid-seventies. His blood pressure was marginally better, although he still looked pale as hell.

"We'll get you more dried off at the hospital."

Slowly, he nodded.

"If I ask you a question, I'm going to need you to open your eyes and talk to me, okay?"

His voice was small, almost like a child's, when he spoke again. "Okay."

I shook my head and looked back at the monitor. He continued to stabilize in transport. By the time we dropped him off at the hospital, we could ween him down on his oxygen so that all he needed was a nasal cannula.

I gave a report and got him moved over to the ER bed. His parents arrived shortly after dropping him off. They both had red eyes and as soon as his mother saw that he was awake, rushed to give him a hug. I noticed the dad, however, stayed on the periphery of the room. It took a great deal of restraint not to walk up to the man and tell him exactly what I thought of him.

But that wasn't my job. My job was to get him to the hospital in the best shape that I could. I walked back out to the ambulance bay where my partner was working on cleaning up the back of the rig.

"Guess you were right about today."

"Huh?"

"You felt a disturbance in the force. Doesn't get more disturbing than that. Do you think that he'll be okay?"

"Mentally or physically?" I asked.

He thought about that statement for a moment. "I guess both?"

"I think we got him here in time," I said. "But I'm more concerned about what his home life is going to be like. What if he's gay? Hearing your parents say something like that can really fuck you the hell up."

My partner shrugged. "You're right, words are dangerous."

Chapter Five

My P****

One of my most feared nemeses during my time in EMS was stairs. They were rarely wide enough or cleaned off enough, or just accessible enough. It was a warm muggy day in July and my partner and I were sitting in an ambulance posting at a gas station. We hadn't been that busy that day, just a few returns to nursing homes. I was nodding off when our pager went off and the radio informed us of a call at a private residence.

Finding the general area of the call didn't prove to be too tricky, however, finding the actual address was more difficult. We circled the block twice before finally locating it. The shrubs at the front of the house had grown so high that you could barely see the front yard and the trees covered most of the upper story.

We got out and grabbed our bag along with the cot. Our first problem was the fact that there were at least four cars in the driveway, half of which had no tires on them. The whole front yard was overgrown with weeds, grass, and a variety of small shrubs and other foliage. What else didn't help was the fact that discarded appliances, boxes, and more cars littered the area. The stairs to the house were covered with debris and trash, and the porch had an assortment of used and rushed washing machines.

"It's going to be one of those houses, isn't it?" my partner asked.

"Yeah, I think so."

We worked our way up the steps to the front door and then knocked. There was no answer to my first knock, but the second time around, I heard someone shuffling around behind the door. It opened just a crack.

"What do you want?"

"EMS, you called and said someone was having back pain?"

"Oh, yes, the ambulance people, come in, please."

As the door opened up, we saw a small, wrinkled man that looked like he was in his eighties. He wore a bathrobe that was splattered with a rainbow of stains and his white hair was sticking up like he stuck his finger in a light socket.

The inside of the house was just as bad as the outside. At least outside there was space for the odor to dissipate. The inside of the house was another matter entirely. There was a powerful odor of cat urine, mixed with the smell of rotting garbage, and weed. It was one of the most unpleasant cocktails of smells that I ever had the misfortune of smelling.

As the man pulled the door open, an entire mountain of newspapers behind him collapsed and only didn't end up on the floor because the door was in the way. Everywhere you looked inside the house, there were piles and piles of trash and just stuff.

Another thing I noticed was the fact that emerging from those piles of stuff were cats. Lots and lots of cats. An unhealthy amount of cats, if you ask me. They all started to meow and crawl around us, much to my dismay.

"Where is the patient?" I asked.

"She's upstairs. It's my wife, you see. She's got a bad back, and it keeps acting up."

"Where are the stairs?"

The man shuffled ahead of us, pushing aside pile after of trash and other debris. The staircase was free of clutter, although the same couldn't be said for the landing at the bottom and the top. My partner and I exchanged worried looks.

"Let's just leave the cot here until we know what we're dealing with," I said.

"She won't be able to walk down the stairs," the man said. "That's part of the problem."

"We'll just have a look at her first."

We slowly made our way up the stairs, trying to avoid the herd of cats that seemed to be determined to trip one of us up. When we reached the top, the man pointed to a door at the end of the hallway, which had stuff stacked ceiling high on either side, with only a narrow path down the middle.

"I know that we have a lot of stuff," the man said. "But we're working on getting rid of some of it. Do you have to report us to the city again?"

"Let's just focus on getting your wife better first," I said.

He nodded. "Okay."

We reached the end of the hallway, and I slowly opened the door. "EMS, can we come in?"

"My back!" she screamed. "Oh god, it hurts!"

Inside the room, there was a woman laying in bed. She was fairly large and, much to my surprise, the room was entirely devoid of clutter and crap. At least it would make moving around in a confined space a little easier.

She was on her back, rolling around and moaning. She looked like she was about the same age as her husband, with matted white hair. The nightgown she wore was, unfortunately, almost entirely see-through because of its age. And just our luck, she wasn't wearing anything underneath. We set our bags down and then assessed our patient.

"When did the pain start?" I asked, as my partner got some vital signs. "Did you fall down or anything?"

"No!" she shouted. "Can you give me something for the pain?"

"I need to exam you first," I said.

I knelt down and noticed several pill bottles on the nightstand. As she continued to roll around on the bed, I grabbed one of the pill bottles and looked at the label. Oxycodone is a fairly potent narcotic pain medication. To make matters worse, there were another three empty bottles for the same prescription. My heart sank for her. Addiction was a serious problem and judging by the date on the pill bottles, they should have lasted her for half a year.

"I can't have morphine. The only thing that works for my pain is something that starts with a D."

I looked at my partner and then back at her. "Demerol?"

"That's the one. It's the only one that works for me."

I didn't even bother pointing out to her that morphine was the same kind of medication as oxycodone.

"Let's get an IV started and once we get downstairs, we can give you something for the pain, okay?"

"Thank you, that sounds good," she said.

"Pain meds?" my partner asked, as I inserted the IV.

"I'll give her some Ativan when we get down the rig. That should help with the muscle spasms."

Getting the cot up the stairs was slightly challenging. We worked on widening the path that was outside the bedroom for a minute or two so that things wouldn't collapse on us as we moved by with her on the cot. Once we secured her to the cot, we left the bedroom. One particularly enormous cat had shown up and seemed keen on following us toward the stairs. I tried my best to ignore the cat, hoping that he might just go away.

Once we got to the top of the stairs, we collapsed our legs, braced ourselves, and carried her down. It was taking all of my concentration not to drop her when I felt something go past my ankle, followed by a strangled meow/yelp, and then a thump. I was not prepared for the words that came out of the woman's mouth.

"My pussy!"

This almost became the first time that I dropped a patient. I had to try really, really hard not to laugh. And then it got worse. Every step that I went down, I ended up kicking this damn cat, who would make the same meow/yelp noise.

"You're kicking my pussy!"

"Sorry ma'am," I said, struggling to hold my laughter in so that we didn't overturn the cot on the stairs.

"Please stop, my poor pussy!"

Dear. God. Make. It. Stop.

"You're going to hurt my pussy!"

By the time we reached the bottom of the stairs, my face was beet red and I was in actual danger of peeing my pants. We pushed her through the main floor and then out onto the porch. It took us another five minutes to navigate our way back through the yard and then down the driveway before we could load her into the ambulance.

As we drove toward the hospital and gave her some ativan. Luckily, she fell asleep shortly after that. Her husband followed us in one of the many cars that he had scattered around the property, although I do not know how he got it out of the driveway.

"So, do you want to tell the ER what you did to her pussy?" my partner asked me from up front.

"You can just shut the fuck up," I said. "We are not telling anyone."

"Are you sure about that?"

"I will kill you and bury you in their yard," I said.

My partner laughed all the way to the hospital.

Chapter Six

Crash

WARNING: This chapter will discuss the death of a pediatric patient. There will be some depictions of traumatic injuries that might be too strong for sensitive readers. I have toned it down some but it will be graphic.

We all have those calls or those patients that stick with us. They change us as practitioners of medicine and sometimes as human beings. This call would forever alter me as a paramedic and a person. It was this call that would force me to re-evaluate my time in EMS. Everything about that day has been burned into my mind.

It had been cloudy and rainy off and on for the entire day. I was nearing the end of a three-day stretch on shift and ready for some much-needed days off. We hadn't been that busy that day and had gone out to the local airport to check the equipment that we used for flight operations. By late afternoon, the rain had tapered off, leaving only a light drizzle behind.

An uneasy feeling grew in me, although I couldn't really put my finger on what exactly was wrong. I chalked it up to the fact that I was just tired. It wasn't long before dispatch sent us for a tiered response with another local unit for a two-car accident on the interstate.

TRIAGE, TRAUMA, AND DRAMA

I didn't have a good feeling about this. I said nothing to my partners, however, as we loaded up and took off down the road, just as rain started to fall again. A gnawing feeling reappeared in the pit of my stomach and I had to force myself to take several deep breaths to stop from freaking out on the way to the scene. I kept telling myself that this was just exhaustion from working three days in a row.

As we approached the accident area, my anxiety grew. That gnawing feeling got even worse, especially when I saw the state of the accident scene. Cars were lined up down the interstate, forcing us to drive on the shoulder.

"Fuck me," I said. "What the fuck happened?"

"Not good," one of my partners said. "Is that the car?"

I saw what was left of a family sedan in the middle of the interstate. It looked like it had almost been sheared in half on impact. The impact had scattered debris all over the road, shoulder, and ditch. The other car was across the road. The front of that vehicle was smashed completely and the front windshield was gone. There didn't seem to be much left of either car.

There were two large tarps over the front of the vehicle. I knew that meant that the people in that car were dead. As we got out of the ambulance, I felt my pulse start to race. I could smell gasoline in the air. It didn't take long before we located our patient, surrounded by a group of EMTs, firefighters, and bystanders that had stopped to help. We found our patient, an 8-month-old, laying on the ground with several people working on them. CPR was already in progress. The look on everyone's faces at the scene should have told me how the rest of the call was going to go. They all looked exhausted and soaked.

"What happened?"

"Crossed the median," the paramedic said. "Got hit and broke the car in half. All the people in the other car are dead. We sent his dad in our squad to the trauma center. It took us a while to find him, he was in the car seat down the road."

The first responding unit had already placed an IO and had gotten a secure advanced airway in place. Thank the gods for small favors on that part.

"Car seat came out of the car and impacted on the pavement," he continued. "Not responding and breathing on his own when we arrived on the scene. We got a tube in place and started CPR."

"How long has he been down?" one of my partners asked.

"Twenty to thirty minutes."

The numbers on out-of-hospital return of spontaneous circulation were not great. Yes, it did happen but it often came with serious damage to the body that would have lasting health repercussions down the road. I looked down at our patient and then back up at my partners. We knew it wasn't good. He was pale. Bruising on their abdomen pointed to possible internal injuries. As bad as those were, though, the damage to his head was much worse.

His cranium was getting bigger by the moment. Spinal fluid and blood were leaking out of his ears and nose. The more CPR we did, the larger his head became. His pupils were fixed. I knew he was dead and even if we somehow got a return of circulation, there was a very high likelihood that he would be in a vegetative state. The monitor was showing PEA (pulseless electrical activity) a rhythm that was just as deadly as asystole (flatline.)

But the longer that we worked on him, the more we all realized that things would not get any better. Despite this, though, we loaded him into the ambulance and took off down the road toward the trauma center, with his mother riding up front. She kept looking back at us, asking if her baby was going to be okay. I kept telling her we were doing everything that we could. She had looked at us with such hope in her eyes like we were exactly like the heroes that you saw on TV.

As we drove toward the trauma center all I could do was think about the futility of the current situation. We worked our asses off in the back of the ambulance, giving him more epinephrine and continuing CPR, even though things weren't improving. CFS fluid continued to pour out of every orifice.

"Anything?" the other medic asked.

My partner checked for a pulse but felt nothing. We gave another round of epi and continued bagging and doing chest compressions again. He continued to leak CSF and blood from his ears, except now it was coming out of her nose as well. His head continued to expand, swelling from a collection of blood from what was most likely a broken skull.

The three of us working on the patient exchanged a knowing look. This child was dead and there was no amount of CPR that was going to bring him back. We all knew he had suffered some sort of catastrophic head injury, not to mention multiple other injuries that were incompatible with life.

The ambulance screeched to a halt inside the ambulance bay. The back doors flew open and several nurses arrived to help us unload the patient. We moved him to the trauma room, doing our best to put on a brave face for the mother of the patient. She was running behind us, shouting questions and asking if he was going to be okay. I couldn't even look her in the face for fear that my expression would give away the futility of what we were doing.

The arrival at the trauma bay was a blur for me. We gave report to the doctors and nurses and as soon as I could, I bolted her from the room. Ran straight out of there like my hair was on fire.

I remember a feeling of overwhelming dread and panic setting in. My heart raced, and I felt dizzy and like I needed to vomit. And then I did vomit. I just stood there over the trash can, my head spinning and my heart pounding out of my chest. Panic attacks were nothing new to me, but I had never experienced one this intense, I started shaking and broke out in a cold sweat.

My partners appeared a moment later, pushing the cot that still had blood and spinal fluid on it. I didn't even bother to ask how it was going in trauma bay, I already knew the answer. A moment later I could hear the wailing of the mother from the trauma bay. That wail, that chilling noise, cut me to the bone.

One of my partners came over to me and slowly steered me to the bathroom. Once we were in the bathroom, I realized I had that kid's blood on my flight suit and even somehow on my face. I just stood there, looking at myself in the mirror, wondering what the hell I was doing. We should have called it. We shouldn't have given that family any false hope.

I splashed some water on my face to calm myself down somewhat. When I came out of the bathroom, I was at least clean, although I didn't feel any better. We said nothing to each other as we got in the ambulance and pulled away from the emergency room. And that's when I totally lost my shit.

I just started crying in the ambulance. I just sat there and kept repeating, "I can't do this anymore." Because my partners rock, they put their arms around me and kept me calm as we drove back to the hospital. I cried the entire way back to the hospital and when we got back, the other team was waiting for us. They took our bags and started working on putting them back together again. My friends took me to one of the open rooms in the ER and just let me cry it out. I was in no shape to go back out there and take care of anyone else. Luckily, it was toward the end of our shift so there wasn't any harm in taking us out of service.

I had seen accidents that were much worse than that, at least outwardly appearing. Accidents were where body parts were strewn across the road, and you could barely make out the outline of a human. This wasn't even the first kid that I had ever worked on, so I wasn't sure why it was affecting me so much. Why was I getting this emotional about a scene that I had worked on so many times before? What was wrong with me?

Once we got back to the hospital, our teammates helped us clean the cot and put our equipment back together again. I waffled between feeling nothing at all and experiencing overwhelming feelings of guilt and anxiety. What I didn't know then was that incident would have a profound effect on me and the rest of my career in medicine.

Chapter Seven

Burn

As we talked about in the previous chapter, I was crashing and burning hard. That last call had done something to me. Never in my career had I experienced such powerful emotions. No one ever imagines themselves as the one that is haunted by the ghosts of calls past. I honestly thought that would never be me. But, after that call, everywhere that I looked I saw ghosts.

And it wasn't just the ghost of that little girl. It was so many others, Patients that died at the beginning of my career kept popping back into my head, creating a constant loop of self-doubt. I started to constantly think that I hadn't done enough. I thought they all died because of something that I had done or failed to do.

I had been doing my job for a long time, long enough that I had seen my share of horrible things. People usually ask me what the worst thing is that I have ever seen. You don't want me to tell you that. And then people say that can handle it and I remind them again that I can barely handle it. You don't want those images in your brain because once they get in there, they never actually leave. They are there every time you close your eyes; they sneak up on you in your dreams, and you'll remember them for the rest of your life.

I've watched family members scream, cry, and lose their minds as a loved one passes on. I've looked into the eyes and seen that vacant stare, the one that tells me that their spark, their soul, or whatever it is you want to call it, is all gone. There's a wail that parents let out when they lose a child and it's a sound that you will never, ever forget. Those in medicine see the worst that people can do to each other every day.

I knew I would encounter some of these things when I went into this career field. I also want to stress that just because we knew we would have to deal with death, dying, sickness, and trauma it doesn't make it any less impactful on the person. I hate hearing from people that 'You knew what you were getting into' and even if we did, that shouldn't minimize our experiences.

They talk about it in class and say things like burnout and compassion fatigue. They tell us to be aware of such things, but the truth of the matter is, most of us just breeze past it. I never gave it a second thought, mostly because every paramedic I saw in training never gave it a second thought. The entire time that I was learning how to do this job, I never once heard anyone actually talk about it outside the classroom. I never asked about it either, too afraid of what kind of label they might put on me.

And because of that I never thought it would happen to me. I never thought that I would be someone that felt that weak. I thought that I would somehow be the exception to that rule. That's bullshit.

We are supposed to be the ones that stand amongst the chaos and never let it get to us. Instructors tell us to compartmentalize and divide our lives up so that everything fits into little boxes. We are told to leave it in the ambulance or the ER. We all know it's not easy, attempting to block out all those images, sounds, and even smells. What we do, day in and day out is not normal. CPR is not normal. Shoving a breathing tube down someone's throat is not normal. Shocking someone is certainly not normal. And yet we normalize these actions like we're answering a fucking email. We talk about them to non-medical people like we are discussing invoices.

For years, this pattern of shoving all that trauma deep down really seemed to work for me. I didn't talk about what I saw or how hopeless it made me feel. I never told anyone that I felt like a total failure every time I lost a patient. I never mentioned the increasing feelings of sadness and depression that I was having every time I set foot in my rig.

But after that call, things got so much worse for me. Those neat little boundaries I set up between parts of my life came crumbling down. Ghosts that I thought I had buried a long time ago kept rearing their heads. There was a permanent heaviness in my heart that settled in after that call. A heaviness that ached with each breath.

I remember pulling away from the hospital after the car wreck and then just sitting there at the stop light, almost paralyzed by the thought of what to do next. Eventually, I started driving home, doing my best not to think about the events that had occurred that day. It was raining again and with each droplet that hit the roof of my car, images of the accident kept popping into my mind.

I had never had flashbacks before but I was literally seeing the scene all over again. I could hear the mom screaming for her child, I could feel the rain on my skin. I could smell the blood and the gasoline on the wet pavement.

I had seen way worse than this. I had witnessed horrendous acts of violence and had walked away without shedding a tear. But this incident tore me up inside. I calmed myself down by the time I got home. My fiance was waiting for me and the moment I walked in the door. He took one look at me and knew that something was up.

He didn't ask if I was okay because he knew I wasn't. He knew that something had broken inside me that day and all he did was give me a hug and tell me I was okay. I once again said I was fine and that I would feel better in the morning. I knew that was what he wanted to hear, what he needed to hear, but I also knew, deep down, that it wasn't anywhere near the truth.

Sleep never came that night, or many nights afterward. The next few days went by in a blur. I stopped eating, I couldn't sleep, and I had zero ability to focus on anything. The closer it got for me to go back to work, the more anxiety seemed to build. I thought it was just jitters and that I would get over it. The night before my first shift after that call, I didn't sleep. I lay awake in bed, images from the side of the road playing in a loop every time I closed my eyes.

I threw up twice that morning before I could even get my uniform on. The drive to work was difficult. I could barely concentrate on the road and by the time I pulled into the parking garage, I was hyperventilating and having a full-blown panic attack. Staring at the elevators that lead into the building filled me with a level of dread that I never had felt before.

Sitting in the car, I started having bizarre thoughts that I had never once had before. What if the helicopter crashed? What if the plane ran off the runway? What if someone hit the ambulance? All these things were running through my head as I walked into the building. A torrent of emotions swirled around inside me as I rode the elevator up to the office. Guilt, panic, fear, and so many more.

By the time I got to the office, I was covered in sweat. Not an impressive look in a flight suit. After checking with the off-going shift, I made my way to the ambulance bay. On the way down to the ambulance bay, I stopped by my boss's office. He took one look at me and then ushered me into his office.

"Are you okay?" he asked.

I stopped and, for a moment, thought about lying to him. I felt broken and useless, and like nothing, I did mattered. Why have all this knowledge and training if people were just going to die? What was the point of all that equipment and all those drugs if they weren't able to save a small child?

"I'm not okay. I can't do this," tears were streaming down my face. "I'm freaking out and I don't know what to do about it."

"Are you safe to be at work?" he asked.

And here was there really scary part. I couldn't concentrate and every time I saw the ambulance, the image of that child would flashback to me. There was no way that I could get back in there and deal with a seriously sick or injured child. Luckily, my boss had been a paramedic long enough to understand what I was going through.

"Do you feel safe to go home?" he asked.

I had battled with anxiety and depression. I had my brush with suicidal thoughts, so I knew what that felt like, and although this felt the same, it also felt different. Every time that I closed my eyes, I would see her face. I could hear the rain falling on the concrete and the vehicles that were parked on the side of the road and could still hear the thunder in the distance.

"I think so," I said.

"You think so?"

"Being in this building and that ambulance, it just feels... wrong to me somehow. I know you want a better explanation, but that's the best that I can do. I feel exhausted already, mentally drained, and emotionally I feel like I'm teetering on the edge of losing it entirely."

"Then I need you to go home."

"We'll be short-staffed."

"We'll figure it out," he said. "I think you need to take some time off if you're feeling that way. I'll send you the links to the FMLA paperwork and the EAP stuff. You can call me if you need to talk."

"I'm sorry."

"You have nothing to be sorry about. You're human."

I nodded, although there was a part of me that wondered if I could ever help anyone again because, at that moment, I seriously doubted my career choice. I felt broken and like I had somehow failed that patient and those parents. Logically speaking, there wasn't anything that we could have done on the side of the road. The damage was done before we even got there.

"I need you to really hear the part about it not being your fault," he said. "Sometimes we do everything right and people still die."

On some level, I knew that, but watching that child die after countless other deaths changed me somehow. I was always told that these things were just part of the job and that I had to be tough enough to endure it. By the time I got back to my car, I was crying again.

The drive back home was surreal. I kept thinking that I was losing my mind, or that I wasn't tough enough. When I got home, I collapsed into bed and didn't wake up for another six hours. When I opened my eyes again, I found my fiance sitting on the bed next to me, gently shaking me awake. He asked why I wasn't at work and then it call came tumbling out.

Insomnia, anxiety, the feeling of dread and numbness. He knew that the last call had been hard on me, but I hadn't told him just how badly it messed me up. We just sat there on the bed, where I cried for what seemed like hours.

Thank god for him, my family, my friends, and my team. I'm not sure how I would have made it through all that without those wonderful people at my side. For the next several months, every time that it rained I would flash back to that scene. The smell of gasoline would start my heart racing and a feeling of panic would set it.

I found help from a therapist that specialized in treating first responders. Confronting those feelings of guilt, anger, and frustration was a harrowing experience. I buried the trauma I had deep, after years of forcing down all the anger, frustration, and guilt I had about my job. It wasn't easy to process most of those emotions, though. I went through so many weeks where I felt raw, like an exposed nerve. The road back would take months and it would forever change me.

I ended up leaving that position to take a less acute role in the hospital to give me a mental break. I couldn't handle another call like that because if it happened again, I wasn't sure that I could come back a second time.

Chapter Eight

Clear!

I talk a little bit in later chapters about shit magnets. Generally speaking, these are co-workers who have some innate ability to summon forth the weirdest and wildest shit while they are on shift. These people, usually by no fault of their own, create an influx of patients, calls, and general mayhem. They don't even need to be EMTs, paramedics, or nurses. I have actually known plenty of doctors, PAs, and NPs that are perfect examples of this.

We had a resident in the ER where I worked that was by far one of the largest shit magnets that I had ever had the pleasure of working with. This poor man would no sooner arrive for his shift than all hell would break totally loose. Ambulances would encode with CPR in progress patients, the waiting room would become swarmed with the weirdest shit that you could ever see. I'm talking about vacuum cleaners stuck on body parts weird shit (use your imagination.)

Since this resident had arrived and started his shift, we had already dealt with a remote in the rectum, an allergic reaction to latex (you can figure out where), an icepick through the cheek, and two meth heads that used frying pans for weapons and literally beat each other senseless. Needless to say, we were pretty busy and our shift wasn't even half over yet. The radio crackled to life, instantly getting our attention.

"Medic 12, coming in hot, code 3, CPR in progress, ETA three minutes."

And then it shut off, without even waiting for us to acknowledge that we heard them.

"Well, that sounds awful," the charge nurse said. "Let's get to the trauma room."

The charge nurse had assigned me to trauma that night, so I ran in that direction. The code team arrived at the trauma room just as the paramedics came through the door. One of the EMTs was on the cot, giving the guy chest compressions while another bagged the patient through the ET tube.

"Fuck me," the resident muttered as he came into the trauma room. "I thought we would be done with this shit by now."

"This is all your fault," I said, as we moved the patient over to our bed.

"He's right," the charge nurse agreed. "You're a total shit magnet."

I took over chest compressions as EMS gave a report. The forty-two-year-old man was found unresponsive in the park. Unknown downtime, EMS arrived and found that he didn't have a pulse, started CPR, and gave epinephrine. No outward trauma was noted, and pupils were sluggish but not yet fixed. No response to Narcan either, so much for making it easy on us. At this rate, the poor resident was going to get a complex with the number of shitty patients that he had.

"Fuck!" I heard one of my co-workers say.

"What?" I asked.

"This line is no good!"

"What about that?" I asked, pointing to his other AC.

TRIAGE, TRAUMA, AND DRAMA

She tried it but it wouldn't flush or drawback.

"Well fuck," I said, echoing her previous statement.

One tech stepped up and tapped me on the shoulder. "I got compressions next. You look for an IV spot."

"Where are my labs?" the resident snapped.

"We're working on them!" a nurse shouted back. "In case you haven't noticed, we're a little busy here."

"I need my labs!" he snapped again.

"Do you want to start the fucking IV? And his labs are going to be shit. Because you know he's dead."

"But I need them."

We were looking everywhere to place another line on the guy. The fire department had tried many times by the looks of it, without a lot of success. Not that it surprised me. The guy had track marks up and down his arms. He was probably a heavy drug user, which wouldn't help our case any. It was too much to ask that Narcan would have worked.

"IO?" I asked.

IO stood for interosseous, which is where we basically put a needle into your bone in order to give you fluids and medication. It actually sounds worse than it is.

"Tried four times, missed every single one," another nurse said. "I'm going to try again but don't count on it."

"Well, fuck me," I said.

I had moved to the guy's feet with another colleague and was looking for any place else to put the IV. We both seemed to find a vein at the same time on each foot and went to work cleaning his skin.

Now, if you've ever been in a trauma bay or experienced a code, you know it is a noisy event. Even when people are trying to keep the conversation to a minimum, there's a lot of commotion going on.

People are yelling things out, someone is probably crying, and you're all focused on getting your specific job done. On this day, it seemed even louder than usual. So much commotion that I didn't hear the defibrillator charging. That is one sure way to get everyone's attention in the ER.

Usually, the sound of the defibrillator charging up would make me jump back from the bed like it was on fire. But that afternoon I tuned it out. It was something that I would never let happen again. The commotion in the room drowned out the sound of it charging up. Before you push the shock button, you're supposed to make sure that everyone is clear by not only yelling it but also by doing a visual to make sure that no one has physical contact with the patient, bed, or anything touching the patient.

What happened next was one of the most painful experiences of my life. I don't actually remember the jolt. The next thing that I knew, I was lying on the floor, feeling like someone had slammed a hammer into my chest. My whole body burned and my chest felt like it had been set on fire. I had never, in my life, experienced that level of discomfort before. The pain lingered intensely for a few seconds and then vanished, followed by the sudden feeling that my heart was about to explode out of my chest.

It was then that noticed two of my colleagues kneeling next to me, chanting my name.

"Are you okay? Can you hear me?"

I nodded, although I couldn't really get my mouth to form words. It was then that I realized the burning sensation in my chest and the numbness in my face. Before I could even try to voice what I felt, they hauled me to my feet, plopped me into a wheelchair, and rushed off to the adjoining trauma room.

"What happened?"

Was I slurring my words? That can't be good. Was I having a stroke? I didn't feel like I was having a stroke, although I had never had one before so I guess I didn't have a frame of reference.

"Idiot resident didn't say clear loud enough for you to hear," the nurse said. "You and Ashley got shocked at the same time as the patient. I'm going to hook you up to a monitor and get an IV started."

"My face feels numb."

"Yeah, you're kinda pale."

"And my chest feels like its... buzzing. And it hurts, holy fuck it hurts."

"Just hang in there."

And then I felt like I wanted to throw up. And then I threw up, narrowly avoiding another colleague of mine by mere inches. Somehow, one of them slipped an IV into me while I was vomiting all over the place. I knew that wasn't a good sigh. What the fuck kind of rhythm was in where my chest felt like this? No way this was a normal rhythm.

"He needs something for pain."

At this point the shit magnet stuck his head into the room. "Is he stable?"

"Yeah, no thanks to you. Get in here and write some orders you dumbass," a nurse said.

That made me smile. At least, I thought I was smiling. My face still felt like it wasn't back to fully working like it was supposed to. The urge to throw up came again and I vomited into a bucket that they had placed on my lap.

"Would you write some fucking orders already!"

The resident looked up at the monitor and then back at me. "Is that really his rhythm?"

"Yup, now write some goddamn orders!"

They must have seen the rather panicked look in my eyes because one of the nurses turned to me and smiled. "We're gonna give you some pain medication, Zofran, and fluids okay?"

I tried to crane my neck to see the cardiac monitor, but they twisted it away.

"You don't need to see that right now."

The fuck I didn't, I knew what that meant and it wasn't good. I tried to furrow my eyebrows at them, but I still couldn't make my face work right. That couldn't be a good sign. When I looked over again, I could see them squeezing a bag of fluids into me. Staff that I had known for years looked tense, the same tense I saw on their face right before we all knew shit was going to hit the fan. I was going to be that guy that was going to crump. There was a flurry of movement at the bedside as a nurse started giving me meds. The shit magnet had ducked out of the room at this point to check on the other nurse. Apparently, they called the code on the guy next door shortly after we both got zapped.

The pain in my chest went away, and I watched some of the tension drain from their faces at the same time. My face seemed to work better after that. After about five minutes, they turned the monitor around so that I could see the rhythm again. Fast but normal.

Everyone in that room breathed a sigh of relief. I actually got off pretty lucky. I came out of the unusual rhythm on my own with some oxygen and fluids. The other nurse that got zapped ended up needing medications and to be cardioverted.

Moral of the story: always make sure the patient is clear before you deliver the shock.

Chapter Nine

Judge and Jury

My job, as a medical professional, is to treat you regardless of your circumstances. That's fairly easy to do when you are treating most of your patients. They aren't the bad guys or convicted felons. At least until. I've had that experience a few times in my life. For the first few, it was hard to take a step back and treat them like any other patient. But this next one, well, he tested every moral fiber of my being.

We were sitting in the dayroom, vegging out and watching TV, when the tones crackled to life over the speakers. A minute later, we pulled away from the station. One of the first things that we noticed that night was the thick layer of fog that seemed to envelop well, pretty much everything.

The call was for an intubated fifty-four-year-old male that was suffering from a drug overdose. We got little more information than that, other than they requested we come with lights and sirens. That was never a good sign.

"We aren't going anywhere fast in this soup," my partner said.

"But they want us code three," I said. "They never want us code three for anything."

"No way that bird is going to fly in this shit," he said. "That's why they want us there so fast. This poor bastard is going to be circling the drain."

I nodded in agreement. It took us an extra fifteen minutes to make it to the facility with the weather. When we pulled in, I noticed several sheriff and police cars, something that wasn't normal. Once we were inside, we went to the ER and located our patient. He looked like death warmed over.

"This him?" I asked.

One nurse nodded. "Yeah, we need this guy out of here now."

That was never a good sign. The faster a sending facility tried to push you out the door with a patient, the worse it usually was, and given how they were already throwing him on the cot, I could tell that this would not be good.

"What's he here for?" my partner asked. "Do you know what he overdosed on?"

"Lots and lots of pills."

I tried to read through all of them, though there were some that I hadn't even heard of before.

"Oh shit," I said.

"We aren't sure exactly what he took, but these were all the ones in his house. Gave Narcan, but nothing really helped. His pressures are pretty soft and his heart rate has been all over the place. Never was responsive. They intubated him right after he arrived. We haven't even sedated him."

"Suicide attempt?" my partner asked.

"Registered sex offender," the doctor said. "They were going to arrest him today for assaulting two minors."

The nurse shook her head. "The deputies showed up to arrest him. They found him unresponsive in his house with the bag of pills right next to him."

"No fucking shit, really?" I asked.

The nurse nodded.

"So, why are we transporting him again?" I asked.

I realized how callous that sounded, but given what he was being accused of, I really didn't care. The thought made me sick and for half a second, I almost refused to take the call. I could always claim that he was too unstable to transport, but everyone in that room knew that was total bullshit. He was critical, but stable.

"No way he can stay here," the nurse said. "Not exactly sure what will happen if we do, we're already getting people calling about him."

"I can see why," I said. "Let's get him moved over."

We got him moved and secured to our cot, along with the ventilator and the rest of his medication pumps. There was a lot, and I had to make a conscious effort not to turn any of them off as we wheeled out the door. While we had been inside, the fog had gotten worse, further reducing our visibility. Even if we drove code three, we would not be making it to our destination quickly this evening.

We loaded the patient up and took off down the road. I did my best not to think about the fact that a child molester was lying in the back of my ambulance being kept alive by machines that I controlled. I looked outside instead and saw the emergency lights reflected in the thick fog that we were trying to make our way through. It was like driving through a damn cloud.

"Do I even want to ask how much longer?" I said to my partner.

"Fog is pretty bad, I'm going as fast as I can. Is he behaving himself?"

"At the moment, yeah," I said. "I could totally change that, though."

"Not our job, remember?"

He was right. My job was to help whoever was in my care, no matter what they did. It wasn't easy, especially when that someone had hurt kids. Instead, I settled back and kept my eyes on the monitor, ventilator, and the various pumps that were feeding him drugs. I'll admit the temptation to shut them off was strong.

As we continued toward our destination, the patient deteriorated a little more. It was small things first; like a minor drop in blood pressure. But, as the miles wore on, things unraveled even more. It was when we arrived at a dead stop that I knew we were in trouble.

"Why did we top?"

"Train."

"Are you fucking kidding me?"

My partner pointed out of the windshield and sure enough, there was a train directly ahead, lazily rolling along the tracks. He was crumping. He wasn't circling the drain yet, but if I didn't do something, he would be soon enough. So, I went back to work, making adjustments and pulling out all my code medications, just in case.

The longer we waited at that train crossing, the more uneasy I became. His vitals started getting more erratic, and I kept having to make more and more adjustments to not only the meds but the ventilator as well. By the time the train cleared, we were firmly trending downhill.

And for a moment, I considered not doing anything. I know that may make me a shitty human being, but the man was a registered sex offender. They were going to arrest him for hurting kids. I might do the world a favor. But again, I was reminded that wasn't my job. If you were in the back of my ambulance, my job was to take care of you, no matter who you were or what you may have done.

So, I went to work, stabilizing him as much as I could as fast as I could. My partner kept glancing up from the front seat as I worked.

I gave him more epi, and another fluid bolus, increased some of his ventilator settings, and did everything that I could do to keep him alive. Which included defibrillating him. Twice.

For the next half hour, I worked my ass off. I went through a good portion of my drug box and had to keep increasing his oxygen to where I knew if we didn't get to the hospital soon, we would run out of O2. I would not let him die in the back of the ambulance. No fucking way. I do not need that kind of karma hanging over my head.

Once my partner told me we were about fifteen minutes out, I called and gave a report. Not surprisingly, no one seemed to really care about him. The charge nurse actually seemed pissed when I told her I had to shock him twice en route. Not that I really blamed her. I was half pissed at myself.

I will never forget the relief I felt as we pulled into the bay at our destination. When my partner came around and opened the back door, he was more than a little taken aback by the mess that I had created. We pulled him out of the ambulance and wheeled him into the ER, right past the nurse's station.

"Where do you want him?" I asked.

"Is that the guy from out of town?" another nurse asked.

I nodded. "Yeah, and I'd really like to get him off my cot before I have to shock him for a third time."

"Let's put him in five."

We happily took him in that direction as several of the staff followed us in. We transferred him over to their bed, pumps, and ventilator. I had never wanted to be out of an ER so badly in my life.

"Shocked him twice, huh?" my partner asked, as we were cleaning up the ambulance. "I didn't think he was going to circle the drain that fast."

"No wonder they wanted him out of there," I said. "I just hope that he lives long enough to stand trial."

"Me too," he said. "You did a good job, though. He seemed determined to die."

"Yeah, you know the rules, though. There is no dying our multiplying in the back of the ambulance, if he was going to die he has to do it in there," I said, gesturing behind us at the ER. "I thought about it though, especially when I had to shock him."

"Thought about what?"

I took a deep breath. "I thought about not shocking him at all. The thought didn't last very long, just a half second, but I thought it."

"I think we all would have thought that," he said. "We have a job to do, doesn't mean that we aren't human."

I ended up saying that same thing to a less experienced paramedic a few years later. It's still some of the best advice that has ever been given to me.

Chapter Ten

Say What

People say the weirdest things, even in medicine and amid an emergency, the weirdest shit. You think I might be exaggerating but talk to any EMT, paramedic, nurse, or any other healthcare provider, and then can probably entertain you for hours about the shit that comes out of a person's mouth.

'We sedate patients for some procedures in the ER, especially when the bone docs must come and gently shove those offending bones back into their proper alignment. The sedatives rarely last all that long, just long enough to get the job done without the patient remembering.

There was one night, the ortho doc had just finished popping the arm back into place of a teenager that hurt it playing football. The whole sedation went smoothly. The ortho doc got the bone realigned and then it was up to me to recover the patient. I had gotten him to sit up and decided that it was probably okay to bring his parents back into the room.

After warning his parents that he might sound loopy for a while, I went back to the computer to continue charting. I hadn't been sitting down all that long when he motioned me over.

"What can I do for you?" I asked.

He looked me up and down. "You know, you look kind of cute."

He wasn't nearly as quiet as he probably thought he was, especially since his parents looked both shocked and confused. I just kind of stood there for a moment, not sure what to say. I ignored it and hoped that he would forget about it when he was back at his baseline. He, however, had other intentions.

"Oh shit, I don't think my parents know I like dudes."

Well fuck.

Now it was going to get awkward. Maybe they didn't hear him, although again, judging by the look on their faces, I knew they heard him loud and clear. I just looked up and smiled.

"The drugs make you say some pretty weird things."

I did not envy the ride home for that young man or his parents.

Fast forward down the road a year or two and we were called out to a residence for what I assumed was an injury. The pager just said, 'Patient fell out'. When we arrived, we made sure the scene was safe and then entered the house to assess our patient.

Our patient was sitting in a large recliner, being fanned by several members of her family. We introduced ourselves and my partner started getting vital signs as I started asking out the patient what happened. What I wouldn't realize until sometime later was the fact that every single firefighter on the scene was smiling about something. It would also take me a few years to realize this should worry me.

"I'm a paramedic. Can you tell me what you fell out of?" I motioned to my partner to maneuver himself so that we could take proper c-spine precautions. "Did you black out? Are you feeling nauseated? Any vision changes?"

She looked confused about my questions, which had me mildly concerned.

"What do you mean? What did I fall out of?"

Okay, now I was confused.

"You said you fell out, what did you fall out of? Did you hit your head or anything?"

"No, son I said I gone done fell out!"

Now, I was really confused. "Right, and I need to know what you fell out of?"

My partner had moved behind the recliner and had manually taken control of c-spine.

I looked around, hoping that someone else in the household could give me some clue what happened. "Did anyone see what she fell out of? Did she hit her head?"

I started looking at her head, trying to see if there was any sign of trauma.

"Nah, man, she said she fell out!"

"What did she fall out of?" I practically shouted. "Come on guys, you need to work with us here. Can anyone tell me what she fell out of and if she hit her head?"

"What, are you tripping, man? She didn't hit her damn head, she fell out."

"You said that! I'm trying to determine what she hit her head on!"

My situational awareness should have kicked in and I should have realized that everyone else in the room was snickering. But, I was a young, dumb paramedic who hadn't quite grasped the ability o read the scene yet. I turned to the woman in the chair and spoke as clearly and as concisely as I could.

"Ma'am, did you fall out of anything?"

"No sir," she finally said. "I got all dizzy and then fell out in the chair."

Well, fuck me. Fuck the assholes in the room with me, who now had to visibly hold back laughter.

"Do you mean you passed out?"

She nodded. "I was watching my shows and I think I got a little too excited. I made it to the chair here before it happened."

"You can let go of her neck now," I said to my partner.

The next time that someone said they fell out, I knew exactly what they meant.

We've all had those calls or those patients where there are dramatics involved. These are the ones that start screaming that they can't breathe at the top of their lungs. Protip: if you're screaming, you can breathe just fine.

We got dispatched to a cat mauling. I shit you not. That is exactly what the caller told the 911 dispatcher. Naturally, my partner and I were curious..

"What kind of cat are we talking about?" I asked dispatch as we drove to the scene.

The only cats in our area that I knew posed a threat to man were mountain lions, and I doubted they would in such an urban area. Stranger things had happened, though, so I supposed it was technically possible.

"Maybe she got mauled by a cheetah," my partner said.

I frowned at her. "This isn't Africa. Where the hell would a Cheetah come from?"

"Maybe the zoo."

"Wait, you think one escaped?" I asked.

She just shrugged, and we drove the rest of the way in silence. We arrived at a fairly normal-looking house, except for what I considered an overabundance of garden gnomes. The police were there as well, looking just as confused as we were.

"Cat mauling, huh?" one officer asked me.

"That's all the information we got as well," I said, raising my fist to knock on the door. "EMS and police, can you open the door?"

A second later, the door flew open to reveal a woman standing, holding a large piece of gauze over a wound on her arm. I looked past her and into the house, assuming that I would see some large feral cat roaming about. I saw nothing but a small orange tabby.

"Oh, thank goodness that you're here! Come in, come in," she said hurriedly.

"You said a cat mauled you?" I asked.

"Yes!" she shouted and then wheeled around to point at the tabby. "Mr. Cinnabon attacked my arm!"

"That cat?" I asked. "That cat right there mauled you?"

"Let's have a look at it," my partner said.

The woman turned to look at the police. "Can't you taze him or something?"

"You want him to taze the cat, ma'am?" I asked.

"No one is tazing anyone," the officer said.

"Let's have a look at that arm."

"It's pretty bad," she said.

"Don't worry, ma'am, we've seen a lot."

We prepared ourselves for what could have been a pretty gnarly wound when she removed the gauze. What we saw instead was a scratch that had barely broken the skin.

"See!" she said. "He mauled me!"

"That is not what you call a mauling," I said. "You also don't need an ambulance for this."

"It could get infected!"

"Doubtful."

"We'll clean it up for you and then you can see your doctor."

"Should I go to the ER?"

"Please don't."

We cleaned the 'mauled injury' and then went back out to the ambulance. Once we were inside, me and my partner busted out laughing.

"You were right, cheetah mauling it was."

Chapter Eleven

I Know

There was a time when I proudly wore tee-shirts and sweatshirts that said things like 'Doing battle with the grim reaper' and 'I'm a paramedic, what's your superpower? Do I regret saying/wearing those things, yes. Would I do it again, also probably yes.

When I was first starting off as paramedic I thought it was my job to save everyone, no matter what. As long as there was a pulse, I had done my job. Nevermind the fact that the person might be braindead.

In the beginning stages of my career I thought DNR was a dirty word. I would litterally cringe everytime that someone said it. I gave no consideration to the quality of life that person would have. I had a very black and white view on death and dying. The nuances and subtles of prolonging life versus preserving life were lost on me at that point my career.

One of the hardest lessons for me to learn in medicine was that not everyone lives. People die. They die every day from trauma, illness, and old age. There were going to be times even when I did everything right patients were going to die. Despite my best efforts, I wouldn't be able to save everyone.

This story happened while I was working in a hospital. Occasionally, the paramedics would float to the ICU and other areas when the need for additional staff arose. Sometimes, being a paramedic in a hospital is akin to being a whore. You're cheap, you're in constant demand, and the hospital (as your pimp) just gives you to whatever department they feel like needs you the most.

There was a patient at the end of the hall that I was helping monitor. The patient was in his late fifties and on a ventilator. He had been battling cancer for the last three years, first in his liver, and then his lungs, and had now moved onto his brain. He had a large family, most of which were mingling outside his room. When they left to go grab some food, I checked his IV pumps and started his other cares.

He looked exhausted, even though he was comatose. I know that's weird to say but it's the truth. People in coma's were always supposed to look relaxed. But not his face, he looked tense, face drawn tight in pain. He didn't look peaceful at all at least not to me. I never bought the fact that people in coma's couldn't hear you. At this point, I had been around long enough to realize that there was plenty that happened in this world that I couldn't readily explain.

The only reason his chest was moving was because of the ventilator. If I were to shut that off, he probably would be able to take a breath on his own, or at least not very many breaths. The only reason his body could sustain life at all was the constant drip of medications going into his veins. As I stood there, I imagined what a conversation with him would be like. What would he say? What would he want his family to know? Was he in pain? Was he scared to let go? Why cling to a life that was only getting worse by the minute?

"I'm tired," he said.

"I know."

"Why does it hurt so much?"

I don't have an answer for him, other than his body is riddled with cancer. It's full of mutated cells that have ravaged every major organ system. I know there's not much time left for him now, no matter how much his family prays. There is no fixing this but I think he knows that. I think that his family knows that too.

"I wasn't supposed to live this long," he said. "I was supposed to go a long time ago, but I tried to stick around for everyone else."

"That's awfully brave of you."

"I don't think they are ready for me to leave."

"I don't think it's up to them."

I know that hits home for him. It certainly hits home for me. My grandma struggled with cancer. Watching her deteriorate from the vibrant women I knew to barely a shell of a human being tore me up inside. She was ready to go at the end, not that I blamed her one bit. I know that I told her multiple times that it was okay.

"There's nothing else they can really do for me, is there?" he asked.

I want to tell him we can keep him alive for a while on the ventilator and the drips, but I know that's not really living. Not in any meaningful sense of the word. I don't think that you can rightly call it living when machines and medications are doing all the work for you.

"I think I'm ready to go home."

I know that too. I can see it on his face. He looks tired. I don't blame him, I'd be tired too.

"They're going to be angry," he said. "They're going to yell and scream and probably say horrible things about you. They're going to say that you should have done more."

"I know."

"They don't understand. Will you help them? They're going to need lots of help."

"I know."

"I'm sorry that I can't tell them in person," he said. "But I really want to go soon. Maybe when my whole family is here. I think that would be better."

An alarm on one pump shook me out of my imaginary conversation. How long had I been standing there? I stopped at the threshold of his room and turned around, taking one last look. On my way out the door, one of his sons stopped me.

"It won't be long now will it?" he asked.

"It's hard to say."

"Do you think he can hear us? Do you think that he's in any pain?"

"I think he can hear you just fine as for being in pain, I think we've made him as comfortable as we can."

"I think I should tell him it's okay if he leaves," he said. "I don't want him to suffer anymore you know. I keep telling the rest of my family that we just need to let him go."

I looked back into the room and saw that peace had seemed to settle over him. "He knows, is there anything that I can get you?"

"No thanks, you guys have been great."

"Let us know if you need anything."

The rest of his family came back soon after that. An hour later, his heart stopped. He had a DNR, so he could pass from this life peacefully, with his family at his side. He waited until they were all back with him. I know that conversation I had with him never actually took place, but I'd like to think that if it had, he would have taken some measure of comfort from it.

Chapter Twelve

Why To Hide Your Lube

We've all had moments where we seriously regretted doing something. This explains most of my dating life until I met my husband (but that's a story for another book.) This story takes place at a time in my life when I was in A) much better shape, and B) still not fully thinking through most of my decisions. I still had the 'I need to be a hero' mentality. Don't do that. It never works out well.

It had been a slow night, and we had just dropped off a psyche patient at the ER. The man thought that he was the reincarnation of Thor, which wouldn't have been that bad, except he was hurling a hammer at people downtown.

Luckily, the pseudo-god of Thunder was a piss-pour shot and missed all his intended victims. We stopped to talk to the ER staff, and I kept glancing at their safe room, which was where they put behavioral patients so they can monitor them. The door was open, which wasn't that unusual, nor was the mumbling coming from the person inside. At least he wasn't swearing at the staff or threatening them. That was a far more regular occurrence coming out of that room.

"Don't mind him, he's just off his meds," she said. "He's actually been pretty cooperative, unlike our friend in room nine."

"What do you mean?"

"That guy is messed up, got wasted at a college party, and then got high on meth."

"Is he behaving himself?" I asked.

"Kept smacking the nurse's ass when he came in," she said. "Thought it was hilarious."

"Oh, so one of those guys."

"Oh yeah, he even tried to run out of the room after being dropped off."

"That sounds like fun."

"We have differing ideas of fun," the nurse said.

"So, you're telling me we're going to be back in a few hours to transfer him to behavioral health?"

"Nah, I think he just needs to sleep it off," she said and then pointed to the room behind us. "That guy needs a psyche bed."

"Has he been serenading you all night long?" I asked. "At least it sounds like he can carry a tune."

"Oh, he likes to sing alright."

"We should probably get back to work," my partner said.

"I am working. I'm doing an outstanding job of holding this countertop down."

My partner rolled his eyes at me. "Do you really want to explain why we didn't have our reports done?"

"Fine, let me grab a drink and then we can go back to the station."

I wandered down the hallway toward the vending machine and got myself a drink. I took the long way around the unit, mostly to prolong having to go back to the ambulance. I had come around the corner when I heard a commotion, followed by another chorus of 'Greased Lightning' and the sound of several people yelling.

I ignored it. ERs are always full of people yelling at someone or something, so it wasn't really anything new. The yelling got louder. So, being the naturally curious human being that I was, I ventured down the hallway to see what the commotion was about. I really should have just gotten my soda and stayed the hell out of it.

As I came around the corner, I realized two things. The first, the guy from room nine, had gotten out of his room and was charging down the hell like some sort of out-of-control farm animal. The second, and by far more concerning, issue at hand was the man was naked. Totally butt-ass naked. And he was not a small man.

For whatever reason, I decided I should try to stop this runaway flesh train. I didn't think and instead just ran toward him. The man clearly had no intention of stopping and we slammed into each other, going down in a tangle of arms and legs, among other things that were flopping around.

And it was then that I noticed an even more interesting thing about him. He was covered in lube. Now, I know what you're all thinking. Where did he get the lube and why in the hell would the hospital have it? We keep it on hand for medical use only, get your minds out of the gutter. This isn't Gray's Anatomy. Why he was covered in it was another matter entirely and, at the moment, not my primary point of concern.

The man was trying to get back to his feet when security came around the corner and rushed him. The man, seeing security barreling at him, turned and ran back the other way, forcing me to make a decision.

Note: I did not say this would be the most intelligent decision that I've ever made.

I threw myself at his lube-covered body again, hoping to slow him down even a little. The impact of my body against his did little to slow him down, and my hands slipped right off him. I scrambled to grab him again and again I slide off like he was made of teflon.

Security wasn't having much better luck and before I knew it, hands, legs, and other body parts were slipping, sliding, and flopping everywhere. The guy wasn't going down without a fight. He was throwing his considerable weight around like some sort of method-out hippo. I remember watching the security footage later and thinking what the fuck was I doing.

The entire time we were grappling with this man, there was a constant soundtrack of Greased Lightning going on in the background. The guy from the safe room didn't even miss a beat and had I not been in danger of being totally squished, I would have been laughing my ass off.

He slid himself free again and tried to back down the hallway. Security tackled him again, finally getting him to the floor and with enough personnel that escape was impossible. Also, most of the lube was on me. And the floor. And the security guards.

I just laid there on the ground, panting and wondering what the hell just happened. I also noticed that the front of my uniform was covered with lube. Not exactly an impressive look for a medical professional. I closed my eyes and when I opened them again; I saw my partner standing over me, smiling.

"What?"

"And what did we learn?" he asked, offering me his hand.

I reached up to grab it and, thanks to the lube, slipped right out of his grasp and landed back right on my ass. He laughed hysterically while I let out a series of curses. I stood up a few moments later, now covered in grime that had formed a unique layer on my uniform, thanks to the lube.

"We better get you back to the station so that you can change."

"No shit, ya think."

As we walked past the nurse's station, we heard the man from earlier. He was still singing Greased Lightning, oddly appropriate for what had just happened.

Chapter Thirteen

Implied Consent

EMS spends a lot of its time caring for people. Sometimes it's a daring rescue. Other times, it's saving people from their own stupidity. As an instructor once told me, people don't call an ambulance because they did something right. That is probably one of the best descriptions I have ever heard of emergency medicine.

We like to think that every call is going to be a heart attack, stroke patient, or even an MVC. That is not the truth, which is a good thing. Can you imagine the kind of burnout that would cause or what kind of stress that would be on the hospitals? Don't get me wrong, there are calls that are definitely high anxiety and high stress but not every call ends with us doing CPR on someone.

Thankfully, this was one of those days where most of our calls had been pretty easy. A few minor injuries, one abdominal pain, and a breathing problem. We were sitting around in our rig, trying to stave off the boredom of another long shift, when the radio crackled to life.

"Medic 11 go ahead."

"Medic 11 I need you en route to 123 Mockingbird Lane, code 3."

"What are we going for?"

"Sending details to your pager, en route at 16:45."

TRIAGE, TRAUMA, AND DRAMA

I remember looking at my partner and being very confused. My pager vibrated a few seconds later. "Sixteen-year-old male, injury."

"That's all it says?" my partner asked.

"That's all it says."

"We both know that can't be good."

"This better not be dispatch fucking with us again," I said.

"I don't think they'd go that far," my partner said. "Especially not if they actually paged it out."

We were both very curious. This should come as no shock to you or anyone else, but males, especially teenage males, do a lot of stupid things. They are not known in EMS for making brilliant decisions, and that is without the presence of any sort of mind or mood-altering substance.

We pulled up to the house, and instantly I realized something was very wrong. First off, all the first responders, police and fire, were standing around grinning like idiots. I knew that was never a good sign. Especially when they were standing around smiling, waiting for us to arrive.

"Upstairs, third door on the left."

"Can you tell us what the hell is going on?" I asked.

"You'll see as soon as you get upstairs."

"I hate it when they say that."

We proceeded up the stairs, wondering what we were walking into. Situations like this could be good, bad, or amusing. Sometimes all three. Once we walked into the room, I noticed two things right away. The first thing I noticed was the fact that there was a shirtless teenager sitting on his bed. The second thing I noticed was the fact that the firefighter standing in the room looked beet red and like he want to be anyplace but there.

"What's going on?"

In my head, I knew this was going to be a case where things were stuck where they were not supposed to be. Imagine my surprise and horror, really, when another hand shot up over his shoulder. It wasn't his hand. It wasn't his arm. I had a distinct impression that this was going to be one of those calls that would be both incredibly uncomfortable and amusing at the same time. I also hate it when I'm right.

Slowly, we walked around the bed, not really sure what we were going to find on the other side.

"Oh, shit."

Yes, I realize that I completely violated rule number five, but given what I was looking at, I didn't really have any other words to describe it. It was one of those things that they might talk to you about in school but that I honestly only expected to see on TV. As I would learn throughout my career, they had to have been getting some of those ideas from real-life situations, like this.

"Is he…I mean, is she…are they? Is that what it looks like?"

The poor girl, who undoubtedly wished she would die of embarrassment, was attached to the young man in a very sensitive spot. In fact, it is probably the most sensitive spot on the male body. All I could do was stare for a moment before I realized I needed to actually do something. I was supposed to be the professional in this situation.

Now, for those of you who haven't figured it out already, let me spell it out for you. She had braces. Those braces were stuck on the foreskin of his penis. Don't ask me how it happened, mostly because I didn't ask either. Three first responders just stood there for a moment, all of us looking at each other, hoping that someone would come up with a brilliant idea.

"Are you ok?" I finally asked.

The girl nodded.

"What's your name?"

"Cindy."

I then turned to the guy. "Are you ok?"

"Not really, man," he muttered. "She's stuck on my dick."

"Yeah, we can see that. What's your name?"

"Jack! Get her off!"

I can appreciate his eagerness to have her removed from his penis post haste, although I was pretty sure just pulling her off would cause a lot of harm. And no guy wants any injury to that area.

"I need both of you to stay calm."

Yes, I realize that was probably a lot easier said than done. I really did not know what to do. I mean, we never really covered this in class. Airway obstruction, sure. Groin injury, of course. But never, ever, in my entirety of training, did we cover a scenario such as this. This kind of shit only happened on TV.

"What the hell are we supposed to do? Seriously, I've seen nothing like this!"

"And you think I have?" I asked.

"I mean, you are gay."

"What the fuck does that mean?"

I shook my head and returned to the problem at hand.

"Alright, I need to get a closer look here."

"How are we going to get them down the stairs?" Jack asked.

"One problem at a time."

I took one look and realized there was no way that I was going to fix the problem in front of me. It looked like they would need to snip the braces wire. We had tools that accomplish such a task, but the skin was wrapped around the wire in a few places. I was pretty sure that he didn't want me to go snipping around in there without knowing exactly what I was snipping at.

"Here's the deal," I said, looking at both of them. "It looks like part of his foreskin is wrapped in the wire on your braces."

Jack turned what I am pretty sure was an undiscovered shade of red.

"What are you going to do?" the girl asked.

"Can you get me a set of vital signs?" I asked my partner.

"On which one."

"Both."

"Has anyone called your parents?"

The kid turned a bright shade of red.

A police officer appeared in the doorway. "Working on that now."

"Oh my god," David moaned. "My parents are going to kill me! Get her off of me!"

He acted like he was going to push her off him.

"Easy there, man, you don't want to do that," I said. "But we're going to have to call your parents, okay? Cindy, are you having any problems breathing?"

"My jaw is just getting tired," she mumbled.

"Well, don't close it!"

"His pulse is a little high."

No genuine surprise there given the situation.

"Jack, how much pain are you in? Scale of one to ten?"

"Eight."

"I guess we could put them both on the cot. We could carry them down."

"I don't think that we have any other choice," I said. "Let's get the cot up here."

It took a few minutes for the firefighters to get the cot up the stairs and into the room. It took us another ten minutes to maneuver them both onto the cot. And then we had to figure out a way to secure them

TRIAGE, TRAUMA, AND DRAMA

that would not cause more harm and make it safe enough to carry them both down the stairs.

One police officer walked over to us. "His parents are going to meet you at the hospital. I told them they were stable, but the manner was time sensitive."

Well, at least that solved that problem. Hopefully, we would be long gone before they got there.

Carrying them down the stairs was more than a little tricky and took six of us. One firefighter had the foresight to toss a sheet over the two of them so that at least they weren't on full display for the entire neighborhood.

We loaded them up, and I started walking around toward the driver's seat.

"Whoa, where do you think you're going?" my partner asked.

"I'm driving."

"The fuck you are. This is an ALS call. You get back there with them."

I shook my head. "The fuck it is not, they're stable. You can handle it."

"No way! That's an airway issue," he said, shoving past me. "You take it. Place he's going to need some serious pain control."

I rolled my eyes and then climbed into the back of the rig. Once we started moving down the road, I did another assessment. Satisfied that all parties were still stable, I pulled out my cell phone and called the ER. There was no way in hell that I was encoding this over the radio.

Once the receptionist picked up, she transferred me to the charge nurse.

"Hey, it's medic 11. I'm bringing you two patients, one with a groin injury and one with airway obstruction, vitals are stable on both. We're about ten minutes out."

"Why aren't you using the radio?"

"You'll see when we get there."

"I swear to god if this is you pranking us again..."

"I wish it was me pranking you," I said, cutting her off.

The ride to the hospital was the most awkward ten minutes I had ever spent in a moving vehicle in my entire life. Although, probably not as awkward as what my patients were experiencing. I started an IV just so there was a line in place and gave Jack a little morphine.

When we did finally roll into the ambulance bay, we took great care in pulling the stretcher out. I kept the sheet on them to maintain some sense of privacy, at least until the ER staff got a look at them.

"What the hell are you doing just calling me up and declaring that you have a patient?"

I turned around to find a very short, very angry-looking charge nurse staring at me.

"Um, look."

I stepped to the side just as my partner pulled up the sheet.

"Oh, my god! Take them to room three!"

After I gave one of the quickest reports of my life, we stepped out of the room and started cleaning the cot. The nurse stuck his head out the door.

"Did you get a hold of the parents yet?" he asked.

"They're on their way."

"Thanks."

We wheeled the stretcher back towards the ambulance bay, ignoring the odd looks we got from some of the staff that saw us come in. Once we were in the bay and out of earshot, my partner turned to me.

"What the fuck was that? Seriously, have you ever heard of that happening before?"

TRIAGE, TRAUMA, AND DRAMA

"Nope, and I hope that we never have to deal with something like that again."

I'd like to say that was the last time in my medical career I had to deal with an injury like that. Sadly, as the years would prove, that wouldn't be the case. Although that was the last time that orthodontics was involved.

Chapter Fourteen

One With The Force

WARNING: This story will discuss the death of a pediatric patient. If you are sensitive to this subject, please skip this chapter.

This incident takes place about halfway through my EMS career. I'd been a paramedic for close to 10 years, so to say that I was getting used to seeing death and dying would be a pretty accurate statement. Although getting used to seeing it was a far cry from being okay with it. In fact, I was struggling with the amount of death that I had been seeing lately.

I should probably also point out that at this point in my personal life, I wasn't an enormous fan of any sort of organized religion. I remember seeing the things that I had in EMS that made me question whether or not there was a God. The constant stream of violence, death, and sickness that I seemed to see made me wonder what kind of all-powerful being would allow this to happen.

No, this will not be a chapter about my feelings on organized religion. I could write a whole other book on that subject. But what you need to know is as I was struggling with my faith and God or a higher power. It was a terrifying proposition for someone who spent a lot

TRIAGE, TRAUMA, AND DRAMA 75

of his formative years in a Catholic school and going to a Catholic church. I also didn't come out until my early 30s and I still held a lot of anger toward the Catholic church and their teachings about LGBTQIA+ individuals.

If there was a god, why did babies have to die? If there was a god, why would he allow human beings to gun each other down in the middle of the street? The most common response I got was that he gave us all free will. People are the ones choosing to kill each other. God had nothing to do with it. I also felt that was a totally bullshit answer. Even if I ignored the violence, there was a disease, such as cancer. Why the hell would he let that exist? No one decides to get cancer.

It was a chilly afternoon in mid-October, and the ER was relatively quiet. I know, I just said the Q word, but for the story, it really doesn't matter. I was just finishing up stocking one room when an EMS call came over the radio. They were en route with a 3-year-old boy who was unconscious and unresponsive. CPR was in progress. They had a line established, but they hadn't gotten a return of circulation so far.

I remembered thinking that we were going to have another dead kid. I also remember being incredibly pissed. This is going to be the third one we had this week. It had not been a pleasant week for us in the ER. Traumas, stroke, alerts, overdoses; They had hit hard us that week.

The patient arrived in full cardiac arrest. I jumped up on the cot and started doing chest compressions as they wheeled the patient into the resuscitation room. He was pale, cold, and lifeless. His parents were right behind EMS. We established a second IV and started giving drugs, while the doctors went to work on trying to figure out what had happened.

There wasn't a lot of information about the actual event. His mom and dad had gone outside for a split second, and when they came back inside, they found him unresponsive on the floor. He wasn't breathing and had turned blue. I knew cases like this rarely turned out well in the end. Out of the hospital, cardiac arrest survival doesn't exactly have great numbers, especially in pediatric cases. Miracles did occasionally happen, but given the way the patient looked, I wasn't holding out hope.

Nothing we were doing seemed to work. We warmed the patient up, gave him fluids, checked his blood sugar, and drew labs. We put him on the ventilator and continued CPR, hoping against hope that we might get something back. But, as the minutes ticked on and we rotated through CPR compressors, we all realized that things were looking bleak.

"Anything?" the doctor asked.

We all exchanged a knowing look, the same thing look we had all given each other countless times before. I remember getting angry the longer we coded the kid, knowing full well there would be no chance for a meaningful recovery. It doesn't happen as it does on TV folks. Even if there is a return of spontaneous circulation, there are often complications from being without oxygen for that long.

There are a lot of bad things that happen to the human body when the body's tissues lack perfusion. There can be damage to the heart, lungs, kidneys, and brain. The person, although their heart is now beating again on its own, may never wake up. Or, if they do, they never return to the same mental capacity as they had been before the incident.

I know it sounds like I'm saying that we shouldn't try. We should, we need to do everything reasonable and within our power as medical practitioners. But, there is a fine line between saving a life and prolonging a life. Sometimes we forget that in medicine.

I remember doing chest compressions on him and thinking this was a waste of a life, that if there really was a God, why would they allow stuff like this to happen? This kid had done nothing wrong, and neither had these parents. Why was this happening again? What kind of fucked up world were we living in? The longer I stood there, the angrier I became.

You've heard of angry driving, angry shopping, and angry working, well I was pretty sure that the tech was doing angry CPR. We would get a thready pulse back, which lasted for about a minute or two, and then the patient would crash again. This went on for at least forty-five minutes, despite our best efforts. No matter how close we came to getting him back, he'd tank.

I could see the look in the parents' eyes, a look of overwhelming sadness and grief. But there was something else. A look of comprehension, of understanding. I think after over an hour; they knew what the outcome was going to be. The mom reached over and put her hand on the doctor's arm and just shook her head. I had ever, ever, in my life seen such a look of devastation on a person's face. The doctor hesitated and looked back at the parents, asking the silent 'Are you sure question'. Both parents, tears now streaming down their faces, nodded.

"I'm going to call it," the doctor said.

I looked into the patient's lifeless eyes and at that moment, instead of feeling angry, like I had so many times before, I felt something different. Even to this day, it's hard to explain exactly what it felt like and hard to put into words. As I stood there in the resuscitation room, heavy with the feeling of sadness and death, I felt peace. There was still a feeling of sadness and grief, but it was tempered by the feeling that we had done everything that we could. I know exactly how weird that sounds, to find peace in death. I felt the sort of calm presence wash over me. Call it whatever you want; god, the force, but whatever that feeling was, it settled deep in my soul.

I knew that deep down me and my co-workers have done everything we could to save that child's life. Sometimes it's just not enough. That's something that's very hard to come to grips with in medicine. With all our technology, all our knowledge, and all our advancements, sometimes it's still not enough. It's a hard pill to swallow, but it's the truth.

I remember putting the room back together that day. There was still a sense of sadness in that room, although that was nothing new. In situations like that, it always seemed to linger for a while. But that feeling of peace settled to persist, despite that. Maybe it was divine intervention. From that point on, I took a less cynical approach to the world. I wasn't ready to throw myself back into organized religion, but I could at least accept that there might be something out there. Something with a plan.

We found out a few weeks later that the parents of the deceased child were both doctors at another trauma center in town. I had always wondered what made them so calmly decide to stop CPR and now I knew. I couldn't imagine having to make that decision. They wrote us a letter about a month after it happened, telling us they were so grateful that we had done everything that we could to save their child's life.

I've often thought about them since that day, marveling at just how full of grace they had to have been to make that decision. I'm sure it wasn't easy, but I'm also sure that they must have had so much faith in something bigger than themselves they knew their child would be going to a better place.

Chapter Fifteen

Stories From Triage

Triage. The mere name sends terror right down people's spines on occasion. Triage is how emergency rooms sort patients and decide who needs immediate medical attention and who can wait. Contrary to popular belief, there isn't an infinite number of staff in the back. We have to prioritize our resources. This means that even if someone arrives to the ER after you, if they are more seriously ill or injured, they will go back to a room before you. We aren't saying that you aren't uncomfortable or in pain, we are saying that it might not be as emergent as you think it is.

I had been out front in triage for almost eight hours this evening. That is a lot of time to deal with people coming in complaining of headaches, cough, congestion, and things that rarely warrant a trip to the emergency room. At around 11:00 p.m., the doors opened, and in walked this 16-year-old with his hand wrapped in a towel. I tried my best not to roll my eyes.

Our registration people, who occasionally displayed more compassion than me, asked him what his emergency was. "Finger injury."

"Is it still attached?" I asked, not even looking at him.

"Not really."

Now, that got my fucking attention. I looked up and saw the kid standing there, with his entire right hand wrapped up in a towel that already had blood soaking through. What was even more surprising was the fact that his mother, who looked as white as a sheet, was standing behind him, holding a baggie. And in that baggie were the mangled remains of what looked like a finger. At least I think it was supposed to be a finger. It looked more like ground sausage at the moment.

"Holy shit!"

Yes, I just realized I violated rule #5.

I scrambled to get him a wheelchair, while urgently dialing the charge nurse's number. I turned to look at his mother, who then promptly passed out.

"I have a complete finger amputation, not sure what the hand looks like. Also, I need a cart up here. His mom just fainted and hit the ground pretty hard."

"What the hell are you doing out there?"

"I was trying to be good!"

Seconds later, the doors to the back burst open and several staff came scrambling out, pushing a stretcher.

"What the fuck did you do?" one of my co-workers asked me.

"This isn't my fault! I'm taking him to trauma one."

"We'll take the mom to trauma 2."

Luckily, his mom had come around at this point and was at least moaning. That made me feel a little better. I met the charge nurse in the hallway.

TRIAGE, TRAUMA, AND DRAMA

"I am never leaving you out there that long again!"

I ignored her and addressed the patient, who now looked like he was going to pass out and slide completely out of the wheelchair. "What happened?"

"Firework exploded in my hand."

"Is it just his finger?" she asked.

The kid must have heard me because he cheerfully added the fact there was a hole in his hand.

"How big a hole?" I asked as we got to the trauma room.

"The room's getting all spinny," he said.

We got him onto the bed just as his mom wheeled by on the way to the second trauma bay.

"Is my mom going to be okay?"

"She's going to be fine, sweetie," one nurse said.

"I should get back out to triage," I said, trying to step away from beside.

"The hell you are," the charge nurse said. "You are too much trouble out there. I sent Clayton out to relieve you. I need you back here."

The docs unwrapped his hand as we placed an IV, drew labs, and did the rest of our trauma orders. When they got the now blood-soaked towel off, well, let's just say that the kid wasn't kidding. There was a massive hole in the middle of his hand. You could almost see through it.

"Um, how many fingers are in that bag?" our ER doc asked.

"One, I think."

"He's missing his pinky and ring finger. Are you sure there aren't two fingers in there?"

I looked at the bag again. "I'm not sure there's even one complete finger in here."

"Where is his mom?"

"Next door," another nurse answered. "She keeps passing out."

Surgery appeared at the threshold of the trauma room.

"I thought it was just a finger amputation?" she asked.

"That's what we thought at first, too," the ER doc said.

"Let's bandage this up and then I'll get him down to the OR. What the hell happened?"

"A firework exploded in his hand."

"Great, where are his parents?"

"Mom keeps passing out in trauma two," the charge nurse said. "I think registration is trying to get a hold of Dad for consent."

The kid went to the OR about fifteen minutes later and we were able to discharge mom about an hour after that once we were sure that she hadn't given herself a brain bleed or anything. Her kid wasn't so well off and although they could save the hand, he lost two fingers and some motor control and sensation. Still, not a bad outcome for someone that had a literal hole in his hand and a finger injury.

It was almost midnight when I got a text from the nurse out front. All it said was 'You have to read the chief complaint on the patient that just checked in'. That was never a good sign. Sighing heavily, I pulled up the electronic medical record and double-clicked on the only patient in the waiting room.

"Wants to be tested for rabies."

Well, that wasn't entirely uncommon. In the area where I live, we had plenty of animals that were capable of contracting the disease to humans. What I was not expecting was the fact that when I opened up the note it said 'Bitten by squirrel five years ago, wants to be checked for rabies'.

Now, I had a what the fuck moment. If the animal that bit you had rabies, you wouldn't have lived another five years to ask that question.

I shook my head and went out to the lobby to call them back to a room. Luckily, we still had a mask mandate in effect, so I could hide my face.

"What's our emergency today?" I asked once we were in the triage room.

"He needs to be tested for rabies," the mom of the patient said.

I paused typing and thought about the most appropriate way to explain to the patient and his mother that there was no way that he had rabies.

"And why do you want him tested for rabies?"

"Because I'm afraid that he has rabies!"

Arlight, well that gave me some sign about how this interaction was going to go.

"Did he get bit by something?" I asked. "And where at?"

"I think it was my finger," the patient said. "But I don't really remember which one."

"And when did this happen?"

"About five years ago."

Again, I stopped typing and looked at the patient and his mom. "So, if it happened five years ago, what makes you think that you have rabies?"

"It kinda hurts."

"I thought you couldn't remember what finger it was."

"I can't. That's why I want to be checked for rabies."

"You don't have rabies," I said, as I typed in the rest of his information.

"How do you know that?" his mother asked.

"Because you get rabies and you die. If you had it, you'd be dead. That's the test."

"But you didn't test him yet," she said.

"He's still alive. He doesn't have rabies."

"You could be wrong."

"I could be, but I promise you this time that I'm not."

"You aren't even the doctor, you know."

"No, I am not, but I have a fairly good understanding of the human body and disease process and I promise you, if had he contracted rabies five years ago he would be dead. It's a fatal disease."

"Well, I still want him tested for it."

I didn't know how else to respond, so I said okay and finished up the triage note before taking him back to a room. Twenty minutes later, I saw them come back through the hallway and then out the exit. I checked the chart and sure enough, no rabies test was performed, though they swabbed the kid for strep throat.

We had been getting ambulances all night long, as well as an influx of high-acuity patients. This means that patients that are complaining of minor ailments have to wait longer to even get to triage. On this night, wait times were creeping up toward three hours, with most people having to wait at least a half to even get to triage. The situation was not ideal.

We had just received our third trauma of the night when I called a patient and his father back to the triage room. Now, I should probably give a little context to this next part. I had been in triage for almost eight hours at that point and had been dealing with pissed-off and bitchy people all day long. I also hadn't eaten or peed that entire time. My ability to tolerate bullshit was fairly low at this point.

As the patient climbs up on the exam table, I asked my triage questions. I try not to let the questions I get asked in triage surprise me. There are a lot. Some ask about wait times, others ask why we aren't moving faster, and some ask if having a fever of over one hundred will cook your insides. It won't. I was not prepared for the father of the patient to look at the rainbow-colored Superman tattoo on my arm and ask if I was a homosexual. In hindsight, I suppose that I could have refused to answer his question, instead, I simply answered yes. He damn near bodily yanked his child off the exam table.

"I want a different nurse to triage him! I don't want him to be influenced by you."

Ah, yes, because I have the power to turn someone gay. I promise you, if this mythical ability existed, I would have had a much more interesting life. You cannot get gay, it's not a foot fungus. I tried to keep the absolute disgust out of my tone when I answered him.

"I'm sorry, but I'm the only paramedic assigned to triage right now. We're incredibly busy tonight."

"Then I want to talk to your charge nurse."

Again, I shook my head. "She's in the middle of a trauma with a very sick patient. She won't be able to step away. I can finish triaging you or you can have a seat in the lobby and wait until another nurse comes out to triage....which should be in about four hours. Your choice."

"We'll just wait then."

"If I don't triage you, then I can't assign your child an acuity number, so you won't be able to be roomed."

"I don't care," he snapped.

"Fine. Have a seat back in the waiting room."

"What? You need to call another triage nurse out here!"

"I already told you, we don't have anyone else available. Please have a seat back in the waiting room and as soon as my replacement comes out here in about four hours, they'll get you triaged. Now, go sit down."

I should point out that his child was in no danger. He was being seen for a cough and congestion, and he was totally stable. The man stomped off with his kid. They waited another hour and a half and eventually left. The best part was two weeks later, he came waltzing in again, saw me, and turned around, walked right back out. Can't say that I was upset by that turn of events at all.

Full moons bring in the crazies. Everyone that works in the medical field, especially emergency medicine, knows this. It's like when someone says 'it's quiet in here'...and then all hell breaks loose. I kid you not, the weirdest shit I have ever bore witness to all happened during a full moon.

It was around three in the morning and I was just getting ready to leave when my charge nurse asked me to triage the latest patient that checked in. I took one look at the computer and groaned. The chief complaint of the patient was 'concerns'.

Concerns could be used for several chief complaints, although mostly for bullshit. I clicked into the chart to see what the nurse out front had typed in. I was not prepared for what I found and then also instantly realized why the charge nurse wanted me to triage them.

I took a deep breath, put on my best caring face, and then mustered all the fucks that I had left for the evening. I went out to get the patient and then brought her back to the triage room.

"So, what is our emergency tonight?" I asked.

"I died."

"What?"

"I died, well, I mean, I feel like I died. I just feel like something is wrong, like you know I died and came back and there is something missing."

"But you didn't actually die?" I asked.

"Maybe not technically, but it felt like I did."

At this point I was equal parts annoyed and concerned, so I went over and started getting her vital signs.

"Do you have chest pain or difficulty breathing?" I asked.

"No."

"Headache, dizziness?"

"No."

"Are you experiencing anxiety or feelings of dread?"

"Not really."

"Then why do you feel you died?"

"Maybe it was the crack."

Ah, there it was.

"What?"

"I did some crack earlier today. I mean, I think it wore off though."

"And did you feel like you died after you had the crack?"

"Does that make sense?"

"I've never done crack, so I don't know. But your chest doesn't hurt right now or anything? You aren't dizzy or experiencing any problems breathing?"

"No, just that I feel like I died or something."

"So, what exactly is your chief compliant?"

"That I feel like I died. Are you deaf or something?"

Clearly, I was asking idiotic questions.

"Okay, so you came to the ER because you feel like you died, after taking some crack, but nothing actually hurts right now?"

"Yeah."

"Got it."

"I mean, I just feel dead inside, ya know?"

Oh, sister friend, more than you know.

But I was pretty sure my dead inside feeling and her dead inside feeling were two totally different things. I finished asking her all the questions that I needed to, before sending her back out to the waiting room. I'd let the charge figure out how to room her, but for now, she was stable and definitely not dead.

"So, she feels like she died but didn't die?" the charge nurse asked me as I walked past her.

I nodded. "Yup, she feels dead inside."

"Did you tell her she was in the right place?"

"You mean because we're in a place of healing?"

That comment came from one of the new nurses to the department, who hadn't yet had his soul blackened by emergency medicine.

The charge nurse laughed at him. "No, because we're all dead inside, too."

I remember laughing all the way out the door at that comment.

Chapter Sixteen
Squirrel In The Box

There are certain stories you just can't make up. I know it sounds like I'm making that up, but that's not true. Very early in my career, one service I worked for had what we call the bariatric ambulance. This ambulance was designed and purpose-built to help transport and care for the bariatric population.

This ambulance had a winch system, and ramps would pull the patient up into the ambulance. This saved our backs and was safer for the patient, reducing the chance that they might get dropped or dumped off the cot. It happened more often than most people services would care to admit.

Thankfully, picking up these patients rarely warranted an emergency. It was usually for doctor visits, or if they were returning to their house or to a nursing home. Occasionally, they would call us to take them from their house to the ER, but it wasn't a more common occurrence. On this day, however, we got a call from one of our regulars.

This patient wasn't all that nice, and most of us avoided going to her house like the plague. She was often demeaning, rude, and very unpleasant to deal with. So when the call came in, naturally, we all tried to pawn it off on someone else. Unfortunately, me and my partner got stuck with it. We loaded up the bariatric ambulance and started driving toward her house. We brought along another unit for moving help, at least until we got her back out to the ambulance.

She didn't live in the best neighborhood, although her family did a decent job of taking care of her house. They usually had the driveway cleared for us and everything out of the way in the house so that we could more easily maneuver the cot inside. That's a far cry from most people who just assume we have forty-five minutes to clear a path through the mountain of junk inside their homes.

It took us a good 5 minutes to unload the bariatric stretcher and get the ramp set up. Then we had to forge a path through the inside of the house.

"How are you this morning?" I asked.

"You guys were supposed to be here ten minutes ago she said. I'm going to use someone else if you don't show up on time."

So it was going to be one of those kinds of mornings.

I did my best not to sign shake my head. "I'm sorry about that. We had some other calls we had to take care of this morning, but we'll get you to your appointment on time."

"You better," she said. "Because if I have to reschedule, it's going to be your goddamn fault. Can you take it easy on the roads this time? I swear to God you guys aim for every pothole there is out there."

Again, I had to resist the urge to say something snappy back at her. Instead, one of my partners grabbed her vitals while we worked on getting her moved over to the cot. Once she was moved over and thoroughly secured so she didn't fall off, we wheeled her out of the house. On the way out the door, she kept shouting orders to her adult children, complaining about the lack of McDonald's that morning.

It was a fairly pleasant day, so we left the back door to the ambulance wide open. Once we got her down the driveway and over the mini cracks in the sidewalk, we hooked her up to the ramp and started winching her into the ambulance. The entire time, she was complaining about the bumpy ride, the temperature outside, and that we wouldn't stop and get her food on the way.

That was nothing new. She gave us a piece of her mind every time that we came to pick her up. If I thought she was mean to us, she was much worse to the nurses at the doctor's office in the hospital. I had seen her make grown men and women cry.

We just finished getting her secured, and we were about to fold up the ramps when I noticed something rather curious. Actually, she noticed it and responded by screaming at the top of her lungs. We seem to have picked up a very curious onlooker. Sitting on the edge of the ramp coming into the ambulance was a small brown squirrel. The squirrel wasn't moving but staring directly at the patient. Given her treatment of humans, I had little doubt in my mind that she might have pissed off the animals as well. My partner went to shoe the squirrel away when the squirrel decided it had other ideas. And by other ideas, I mean jumping into the ambulance.

My patient shrieked and started thrashing around the cot. After checking to make sure that she wasn't having a seizure, I addressed the elephant; I mean squirrel in the room.

"Where is it?" she demanded.

"Ma'am, I'm going to need you to remain calm," I said.

"You can shut the hell up!" she snapped. "It's going to bite and then I'll get rabies and soon your ass!"

I decided not to tell her that rabies was fatal.

"Where is it?" my partner asked. "Did it run out?"

"I don't see it!"

"You need to find the damn thing!" the patient screamed. "I'm not kidding! I will sue your ass!"

You'd think finding a squirrel in an ambulance would be easy. There really aren't that many places for one to hide, and the back of the rigs weren't that big. Just as I was about to look under the cot, the squirrel bolted out and clawed its way up the cargo webbing. Our patient, who looked back, saw it and started screaming again.

This time, though, she started thrashing around someone that was being tazed. She started ripping at the seatbelts and screaming at the top of her lungs. The squirrel just looked at the shrieking woman and chittered away at her like they were having an actual conversation.

"It's going to give me rabies! Help, help!" she screeched.

"Calm down!" I snapped.

At, that point she was throwing her considerable body weight around so much that the entire back of the ambulance was shaking. My partner and I tried to calm her down, but she continued to panic and the squirrel just continued to sit there. I would have thought the hysterics coming from our patient would have scared it off, but it was just hanging out.

My partner, for reasons totally unbeknownst to me, tossed a gauze roll at it. It had the intended effect of dislodging the squirrel from the cargo net, causing it to fall to the floor. My partner swore and jump up onto the bench seat. This caused our patient, who calmed down only slightly, to thrash wildly again.

The squirrel was running around on the floor, desperately looking for a way. I had moved to the other side of the rig and was trying to shoo it away when it advanced toward us again, and that's when all the moving and bouncing around caused the cot to come out of its mounting and shift directly toward me. With a bariatric patient on it.

Luckily, the cot didn't have very far to go. Unluckily, it was still heavy enough to cause a considerable amount of pain to explode from my ankle. I got pinned between the cot and the rig. I shoved the cot off me, which resulted in me nearly causing her to roll off the cot onto the floor. My partner, still from his perch on the bench seat, had finally chased the rodent from the back of the rig and out the door.

Now, we were all a sweaty mess and the back of the ambulance looked like some sort of war zone. Gauze rolls, tape, and the entire contents of the IV (not sure how that came loose in the scuffle) were all over the floor. In the chaos, and no doubt because of all the arm flailing, she had knocked the tray off the counter area that held syringes, needles, and a few other things.

She burst into tears, screaming about how she was now going to have PTSD. I hobbled around the cot and to where my partner was sitting on the bench seat. Between the two of us, we got her calmed down enough that we could get her buckled back in.

"We should get going," I said. "We don't want you to be late for your appointment."

She almost looked like she was going to protest, at least until my partner got out and went around to the front. On the way to the doctor's office, I worked on cleaning up the back of the ambulance and when we arrived at her doctor's office; it didn't resemble the streets of a combat zone. We unloaded the ramp parts and then brought her into the office.

My ankle was pretty big, and I was hobbling around. We dropped her off. She would be there for several hours and then went back to the ambulance.

"Are you okay?" my partner asked, as I limped toward the front.

"I think so," I said. "Also, what the fuck, man? It was just a squirrel!"

My partner shook his head back and forth. "No way those things carry rabies."

"They do not carry rabies," I said.

"They carry rabies!"

I rolled my eyes. "Okay, if they carry rabies, it would look sick. That squirrel did not look sick.

"Whatever, man, it wasn't worth it. We aren't going back to pick her up?"

"Oh hell no," I said. "We are going back to the station to fill out the paperwork for work comp and then I am going to ice the fuck out of this."

Chapter Seventeen
Shit Magnets

One of the best things about emergency medicine is the people that you get to work with. Whether it's your partners in the ambulance or your cohorts in the ER, they become extensions of our families. They are there in the trenches with us. They've seen what we've seen and can often offer us advice and solace that our loved ones can't.

Some of my favorite people in EMS were, simply put, shit magnets. As much as I liked them, these people were the sort that seemed to have an innate ability to offend the EMS gods and open the gates of hell whenever we would work together. I know some of you may think that I might be a tad dramatic, but I'm serious. Some of the best partners that I've ever had were constant magnets for the strange, obscene, and downright bizarre.

I remember one night; we had gotten our asses kicked. Truly so hard that after our last call, on the way to fuel up the ambulance, I just looked at my partner and said, "Tree pretty, fire bad," which summed up my mode of thinking for the evening.

While my partner started fueling up the ambulance, I went inside to get something to drink and to keep myself awake to author the six ALS reports I had waiting for me. When I came back out of the gas station, I noticed that the back of our rig was open. I was going to commend my partner for his diligence in cleaning the back of the ambulance, especially since the last call left it looking like a bomb went off in there.

As I walked around to the back of the ambulance, I heard him talking to someone. I poked my head around the corner to see that he had someone sitting in the rig and was hooking him up to the monitor. I exhaled loudly, which got his attention.

"What are you doing there?" I asked.

"This gentleman approached me and said that he was having some mild chest discomfort," my partner said. "He wanted to know if we could check him out."

I sighed heavily and resisted the urge to roll my eyes. All I really wanted to do was go back to the station, finish my reports, and try to lie down for at least a few moments before the sun came up. Apparently, though, we hadn't sacrificed enough pagers to the gods of Motorola for that to be the case.

"Sure, why not?"

I stood at the back of the ambulance, sipping my soda, and listening to my partner converse with the man that had climbed up into the back of the rig. I refused to call him a patient. I was just about to walk inside and grab a candy bar when my partner started gesturing at me to get in the back of the ambulance. Actually, gesturing wildly might have been a better way to describe it.

I rolled my eyes and climbed in, plopping myself down on the bench seat. "What?"

"Tell Matt what you were just telling me."

"I had this operation a few months ago, and they told me that if my chest ever started feeling weird, I should go get checked out."

I had a feeling that my plans for the rest of my shift being calm were about to go completely out the window.

"Do you want to show him your scar?"

The man turned to me and opened up his shirt, where I saw a scar that ran down the middle of his chest. And not a faded scar, but one that only looked a few months old. It was then that my partner gestured for me to look at the monitor. I should have never looked at the monitor.

When I turned my head to see what the fuss was all about, I did a double take at the monitor. I did not know what rhythm the man was in. It looked vaguely like it was some sort of weird sinus irregularity (sinus is your normal rhythm) with elevated T waves. My partner, who had been staring at it longer than I had, tried to make a gesture toward the monitor that wouldn't be obvious to our soon-to-be patient. I frowned at him and then looked over at the screen. And then had to work really hard at controlling my non-verbal reaction.

"And yes, the leads are on in the right place," he said.

Fuck. My. Life.

"Does your chest hurt right now?" I asked.

Please, for the love of all that is holy and pure let him say no.

"It's not really pain, just more or less discomfort. It kinda feels like an elephant is sitting on my chest or that someone is trying to squeeze it."

Fuck me sideways.

"Do you think you can make it to the hospital?" I asked.

"I think so. The pain isn't that bad."

My partner, again much older and wiser than I, gave me that look that told me I should probably stop talking and start driving.

"I think we should probably take you to the hospital," I said. "And I think we should probably get moving. Let's throw a line in him real quick."

My partner got to work on a line while I shut the doors and started the rig. Dispatch was a little confused when I called them and asked them to create a trip number for us from the gas station to the hospital.

When we arrived at the ER, the charge nurse just shook her head and directed us to a room. "I should have known it was you two."

"This is not my fault," I said and then gestured at my partner. "He's the one that found the guy."

We dropped the patient off in his room and then went out to clean up our stuff. On the way out the door, we walked by the nurses station.

"Stop finding patients," the charge nurse said. "Really, if you encode again with a patient report, I am going to totally ignore you."

I jerked a thumb over my finger. "Tell him that!"

She just shook her head and went back to work. We did eventually stop bring them patients that morning, just not as soon as the charge nurse would have liked. Turns out that we weren't the only service finding them either.

As we pulled away from the hospital, we saw a gentlemen staggering down the straight. He coul've have just been drunk or he could have been in some sort of distress. It was hard to tell from our vantage point. My partner was reaching for the radio when I swatted his hand away.

"No. Just no. If he needs help, he can call, just like everyone else."

My partner laughed. "Killjoy."

It was an early afternoon during the spring and we were on our way to the store to pick up food for the station meal that evening. We had stopped at a stoplight, minding our own business, when a young man walked across the crosswalk in front of us. No sooner had he gotten in front of the ambulance, that he dropped to the ground like a sack of potatoes.

At first, we thought he might just be joking. So we didn't get out and check, but after he didn't pop back up, and seeing as how were in an ambulance, we decided we might want to look at the situation. We got out and went to the front and found the man lying on the ground and seizing.

"Do you think we can just drive around him?" my partner asked.

Although I hate to admit it, I had similar thoughts. Instead, my partner got back into the ambulance and radioed dispatch. I went to the back and grabbed our gear. By the time we got back to the patient, he had stopped seizing and was coming back around.

He was more than a little surprised when he opened his eyes and found me and my partner kneeling over him.

"What's your name I?"

He just stared blankly at me for a moment and then finally said. "Josh."

"Do you have a seizure disorder?"

He slowly nodded.

"Do you take any meds for your seizures?" I asked.

He nodded again.

"Did you take them today?"

This time you shook his head no.

My partner had him hooked up to the monitor and was getting a c-collar on him. has vitals were pretty normal, so we got him transferred to the cot and then got him in the back of the ambulance. I started a line, checked his blood sugar, and then started the saline bolus.

"Do you remember what happened?" I asked.

"I think I was going to the store," he said. "But I haven't been able to get my meds for the last few days, so that's why I didn't want to drive."

Well, at least he was smart about that.

The rest of the drive to the hospital was pretty uneventful. He continued to improve, and by the time we got to the ambulance bay, he was awake and alert. We dropped him off and then drove back toward the store again. Luckily, this time we made it with no interruptions.

This last story comes from me and an entirely different partner than the first two. We had been dispatched for a rollover accident at around 1:00 in the morning. We were the first ones on the scene on a very dark and freezing October night. There were no streetlights on this road. It was gravel road just out side of town that was full of curves and bends. Those traveling at excessive speed often lost control in the corners, resulting in all manner of crashes. We hadn't come across any debris or the car yet. There were no street lights either, so we were searching with our headlights and the search light in the ambulance.

Cornfields surrounded the road on either side, so we assumed it would be easy to find a car that left the road. As we drove slowly down it, waiting for the cops and the rest of the rescue to arrive, we couldn't seem to find any sign of the accident.

"Are you sure we're in the right place?" I asked my partner.

"This is exactly where we're supposed to be," he said. "Shouldn't we have seen it by now?"

"I think so. I mean, he said he rolled it. That would be pretty hard to miss."

We turned around at the end of the road and came back when we spotted someone emerging from the cornfield like someone that aliens had kidnapped. He was in a torn-up jacket, blue jeans, and missing a shoe. He walked with a slight limp and had some lacerations on his face, but otherwise appeared uninjured.

"I think that must be our guy."

We stopped the ambulance and quickly approached the patient.

"I'm fine," he said. "Just rolled my car back there."

"You rolled your car? Are you the one that called in the 911 call?"

My partner was moving to secure his c-spine when he looked over at him. "Please don't touch me, I'm fine, really. I actually don't really want medical attention."

"What?" I asked.

"You were going to hold my neck still. I don't want that. I'm fine."

At that point, he failed all his limbs about to illustrate that everything worked. My partner and I exchanged a worried look.

"Then why did you call 911?"

"Because usually when I do this, the car starts on fire."

"Usually when you do this?" I asked. "You've done this before?"

"Lots of times."

"Sir, you rolled your vehicle. I think you need at least need to get checked out," my partner said.

The man shook his head. "I'll be sore for a few days, but nothing hurts like it's broken."

"You experienced significant trauma. I really think that you should at least get checked over."

"I'll be fine."

"How did you get out of the car?" my partner asked.

"Crawled out the window. What can I say? I'm not an excellent driver."

"Where's your car?" my partner asked.

The man turned around and gestured vaguely behind him to the cornfield. "It's somewhere over there. Usually, it's on fire by now."

"Your car is on fire?" I asked.

"I don't think it's totally on fire yet. But it's probably smoking. You guys should call the fire department."

"They should be here any minute," I said.

In the distance, I could hear more Sirens signaling the police and fire units. I looked over at the man again.

"I really, really think you should come with us to the hospital. You could have serious internal injuries."

"I'll be okay. Can I just sign one of your forms?"

My partner and I looked at each other. "I mean, we can't take you against your will."

"I mean, don't we have to sort of take him?" my partner asked.

"Not if he's appropriately oriented."

The man then rattled off the date, time, place, month, and year.

"There goes that idea," I said. "So, yeah I guess we give him the form."

"Really? We can't take him in."

"He said he doesn't want to go, not much we can do after that."

"He could be seriously injured! He could die."

"He could, but he doesn't want to go."

"Why is he not boarded and collared?" a firefighter asked. He sighed heavily when he saw who it was. "Oh, it's you."

"You know him?" I asked. "And he's done this before?"

"Lots of times," the firefighter said. "Where's your car Terry?"

The man gestured behind him. "Over there. I don't think it's on fire yet."

The firefighter nodded and then jogged off toward the rest of the department. At this point, a police officer had walked over, surveying the area with his flashlight.

My partner shook his head. "He just rolled his car. We have to take him in. We can't just not, can we?"

"If he doesn't want to go, then we can't take him anywhere," I said. "There was no one else in the car with you?" I asked.

"No."

"I told you, I'm fine."

"He says he's fine."

"Can he do that?" the officer asked.

"He's not altered, so yeah, I mean he can do that."

"Are you sure?"

"Yeah, I'm sure. Unless you need to arrest him for something, there's not a lot that we can do about it."

At that point, my partner pointed behind us to the field where we could now clearly see there was a fire. We both assumed it was his car, and the man turned around to look at it, shrugged, and then turned back to us.

"Can I go now?"

We looked at the officer. "I think he has questions for you but, I mean as long as you don't want medical attention, just sign here."

He signed the paperwork and then walked off with the officer.

"What the fuck was that?" my partner asked.

"I have no fucking idea. Dispatch is going to love this."

Chapter Eighteen
Nope, Still Dead

I know that it's hard to believe, but I used to be quiet and soft-spoken. Those of you that know me now can stop laughing. This story takes place shortly after I started my career as a paramedic. The first few weeks on my own were relatively uneventful. I had the occasional sick patient, but nothing that was too taxing or too complicated.

When you are brand new to a career field, like EMS, you crave the exciting stuff. The stuff that you see on TV or hear about on the nightly news. I'd like to say that I was different in that aspect, but that wasn't the truth. I was young and dumb and yearned for excitement. I wanted the calls that made my pulse race and that would require me to do all the exciting and lifesaving skills I had learned. Codes, an MCI, something other than a taxi ride to another facility. Here's a tip for you youngsters out there: never, ever, wish that something exciting would happen. You wish for dull nights where nothing happens, and you get to finish an entire season of the latest binge-worthy streaming show.

Our pager told us he was on a cardiac monitor, had several drips running, and was on a ventilator. It wasn't as exciting as a three-car pileup, but it was better than sitting around the station doing nothing.

The station was right across the street from the hospital, so getting to the patient was easy and quick.

I should have known that things were going to go all pear-shaped when the unit receptionist practically threw paperwork at us when we walked into the unit. The second thing was the fact that when we entered the room to get report, the RN in the room was already turning off the monitor and motioning for us to hurry. If that happens to you, know that is not a good sign.

"Um, is everything okay?" I asked.

"Yes, it's fine."

"Why are you turning that monitor off?" my partner asked.

"It's fine," she said. "Do you want a report?"

"Yeah," I said. "And where are we taking him?"

"Cardiac floor," she said.

"Assuming he even makes it there," said the tech.

That caught my attention instantly. "What does that mean?"

"Oh nothing, he should be fine."

"I don't like that," my partner said. "Why would he say that?"

I just shrugged and assumed that the tech was just talking out of his ass. The nurse finished giving me a report while my partner transferred over the drips and got him on the ventilator. After securing the patient to the cot and making sure that he was tolerating the ventilator, we walked out of the room and toward the elevators. We stopped and let the family say goodbye. I can still remember his wife's face to this day. She seemed calm and not at all apprehensive. She walked with us to the elevator and gave him a kiss on the forehead.

"You'll take good care of him, won't you?"

"I'll do my best," I said.

"He's in good hands, ma'am," one of the floor nurses said.

And I really thought that he was. I wasn't overconfident in my skills, but I thought for sure that I could handle a stable patient for the quick and easy forty-five-minute drive to the other hospital. Since he was stable, we opted not to transport him with lights or sirens.

However, as I was reading the bible that was his chart, I came across some rather curious pieces of information. Runs of ventricular tachycardia (an arrhythmia with possibly deadly consequences), soft blood pressures, and a generalized tendency to take a turn for the worst with no warning. I checked his vital signs and my equipment. No change, still stable.

I briefly thought about telling my partner to upgrade to code 3, which would have had its own set of dangers. You turn on lights and sirens and every on the road suddenly becomes an unpredictable loon. Besides, he was still stable…for the moment. The more that I sat there in the back of the rig with him, the more I realized something wasn't right. I couldn't exactly put my finger on it, but something felt off.

I was about to learn a very important lesson in trusting your gut. If it feels off, then it probably is off.

As we traveled down the road, I kept a close eye on his vital signs. About twenty minutes before we reached our destination, things went south. I noticed his vitals were trending in a direction that wasn't good. I upgraded to code three after that. No sooner had I said that did shit really hit the fan. He lost his blood pressure completely, and I watched his heart rate go from a steady 70 beats a minute to nothing.

One good thing about having ventilated patients is at least you already have the airway secure. I started compressions, all the while shouting at my partner to find the nearest ER and radio them we had a cardiac arrest. This wasn't supposed to be happening. He was supposed to be stable. Hell, I had told his wife that I would take care of him and he would arrive safe and sound. Now, that was defiantly not going to happen. Safe and sound were out the fucking window.

My partner, thank God for his ability to safely operate an emergency vehicle, promptly stepped on it. He informed me we were three minutes out from the nearest ER. I knew those three minutes would feel like an eternity. My partner gave them a very brief report over the radio as I pushed more epinephrine through my patient's IV line and made sure that his fluid was flowing wide open. After that, I went back to performing CPR on my patient.

It felt like an eternity. I was a sweaty mess as we pulled into the hospital. My muscles burned and ached with the effort of continuing CPR. Luckily, as the back door opened, I saw several ER nurses waiting for me. I had never been so happy to see anyone in my entire life. One of them jumped in and took over CPR as I pushed another round of epinephrine.

We pulled the cot out, and I disconnected the vent to bag the patient. Once we entered the trauma room, I gave a report the best that I could and informed them that the patient's family was already en route to the original destination. I felt like a total idiot the entire time that I was giving the trauma staff report.

I remember walking out of the room, sore and sweaty. I met my partner outside the room, an EMT that had a great deal more experience than myself. He patted me on the back and told me I did a good job. Although looking back through the trauma door, I felt like it had done a totally shitty job. If I was good at my job, then this guy would still be alive and not have someone pounding on their chest.

I went back to the ambulance bay with my partner and cleaned up the back of the ambulance. The news of what happened reached my manager. Oddly enough, he had been at that hospital teaching a CPR class. When I got back from dropping off another round of sheets, I found him standing in the ER bay, talking to my partner.

"How is he?"

"Oh, he's still dead!" I said. "And I don't think that he's getting much better."

My manager smiled. "Yeah, I think you're going to be fine."

We finished cleaning up and jumped back on the rig. I never got to tell that poor woman what happened, although the ER staff assured me they told her that everyone did everything they could to save her husband's life. Still, that was the first time on my own that I lost a patient.

I felt kind of numb like I should have been more upset by the turn of events. The weird part was that I felt nothing at all. We went back into service and never spoke about it for the rest of the shift. It would be years later before I realized just how much that first incident impacted me.

www.ingramcontent.com/pod-product-compliance
Lightning Source LLC
Chambersburg PA
CBHW031436210526
45464CB00005B/2222